GLUTEN: THE ENEMY WITHIN

A timely exposé of all the lies about GMOs

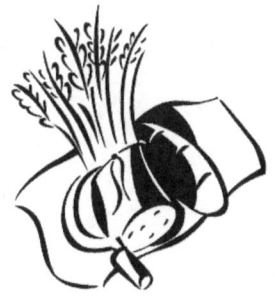

CYNTHIA GALLANT-SIMPSON

BELLY, BELLY, WHO'S GOT THE BELLY?

When all else had failed in my battle against the unwanted belly fat on my otherwise fairly slim body I was tempted to simply accept that mid-life brings changes that must be accepted. However, my intuition kept hammering away at the back of my mind insisting that this was a defeatist attitude. Find the answer, it hollered at me.

My intuition has rarely let me down. We are old friends who have faced many a battle together and won by working cooperatively; a happy medium of analytical thinking and just plain gut common sense. But where to begin to find a solution to paring down that pesky belly that dieting and exercise had not accomplished. I looked around at my mid-life and older friends and then at the general public. The American belly situation did not look good.

Beginning with the premise that my belly fat was an anomaly since I had slim arms and legs, etc. I found that other women of my general age who were slim were carrying around frontal pouches from small to large, as well. What was I missing? What were they missing? I refused to believe that this situation was an inevitable consequence of ageing, post-menopause or improper diet. My diet was fine and as it turned out from talking to a few women about their diets, they had all clearly gotten the message about sugar and fat. They, like me, were practicing safe eating. A discussion arose among a few of my female friends about their husband's bellies and although many of them worked out and ate a similar diet, they too were carrying around more flab than they wanted to on their bellies.

The next step was to broaden my study to the general public. This brought a huge awakening. We all have heard and probably used the term "beer belly". However, how many babies and toddlers do you know who guzzle beer regularly? In addition, how much beer would it take for teens to become seriously overweight, do you suppose? No, beer was definitely not the only belly type.

It did not take long to appreciate the full impact of something I had been seeing in the general public for some time. It merited a much closer look. Egotistical concern about my disappeared waistline and frontal pouch began to seem insignificant when I looked around and realized that from babies to the elderly, right across the board, socioeconomically and racially, people are grossly overweight in our society. Why? When did it begin? I realized that I had been aware of it for some time however, it had remained in the periphery of my consciousness to some extent.

Something so widespread and invasive that had inserted itself into the population at-large called for a closer look. Not to say that I was not aware of all the media hype about fast food, sugary snacks, poor eating habits and soda.

I have been fully aware because one would have to live under a rock not to be. Television has made millions by exposing overweight people to shame and ridicule to film a show called the Biggest Loser. Of course, when the winner is heralded then at least one overweight person achieves celebrity status.

I could only assume that all the overweight people out there of all ages are not beer guzzlers or post-menopausal women cursed by the god of vanishing waistlines.

Certainly, when you see an entire family that is grossly overweight the reason cannot be overconsumption of beer. And there are entire families carrying around dangerous extra pounds. I know the mantra: People eat too much, drink too much soda, eat the wrong things like donuts and other sugary snacks, and gorge on fast food. I have no argument with that proposition. Just stand behind a few family shoppers in the supermarket checkout line and the evidence is appalling. When did soda become the new water for one thing?

Yes, maybe these dangerously overweight people chose to tune out on the advice of doctors and spokespeople for the FDA, American Heart Association, the Mayo Clinic, CNN Health Watch and others concerning the dangers of sugar, salt and fats. No one argues that going cold turkey from your favorite foods is fun. So, maybe some people have chosen obesity over good health. Maybe.

Alternatively, maybe the problem lies in what passes for food today.

The American diet is in really bad trouble.

That fact can be observed anywhere we go where there is food involved. From market shelves to fast food restaurants to the added sections in pharmacies to make sure that when you pick up your prescription for your diabetes or hypertension or arthritis that you can pick up some tasty snacks and/or soda at the same time. By the way, diet soda is just as deadly!

Supermarket shelves are laden with "stuff" that people believe is food. However, the era of food products as opposed to real food is upon us and growing more dangerous every day. I stood laughing so I would not cry when I came upon an aisle in a supermarket designated by the overhead sign as "nutritional food". In fact, it was not a full aisle just a partial where "whole food" was located. Except for the aisles of paper products, soaps, cosmetics and such there were about fifteen additional aisles where "food" lined the shelves but I could only assume that it was designated "non-nutritional" food although I could not find the sign.

Back when people ate real food, markets were smaller. For good reason.

Far too many entire families today are struggling with excess weight. Certainly, there are some who are complacent about their weight, choosing to live with it; it is what it is. However, you can be sure many overweight people would like to shed the weight. In fact, there are those who are perplexed as to why they eat as the government guidelines recommend and still carry all that excess fat around.

Across the nation, there are victims of obesity who got there for the clear and simple reason that they stuff their faces with "bad" food, every day. You know, thick shakes, huge cheeseburgers, giant-sized Cokes and Twinkies. Indisputably, the food choices of a large segment of the population are inclusive to what they see advertised on television, and what sits on the grocery store shelves, prettily packaged and presenting itself as good food. The foods in the middle aisles of grocery stores as opposed to the outer aisles where the "real" food presents itself.

The twentieth-century's great boon to the family cook, habitual snackers, and always-hungry teenagers, quick and easy processed "frankenfoods", are most certainly high on the list of culprits responsible for the nation-wide obesity plague. However, perhaps there is something else on the grocery shelves, hiding in plain sight, disguised as a mighty and unassailable hero of sensible dietary choices.

Yes, we all know the advice about eliminating or at least downgrading our intake of sugars, fats and salts. But might there be something else hiding in this mystery that because of its clever disguise as "good" food is undermining the diets of millions and guaranteeing that they hold onto the unwanted weight?

There is another kind of hype that makes victims of the innocent when they walk up and down supermarket aisles. It calls to them from well-designed disguises. It cleverly appeals to their busy lives by promising to add time and remove a lot of the work entailed in mealtime preparation. How can busy people resist such clever entreaties?

Hoorah for the wonderful new foods that the food producers brought to us in the middle of the century. They promise quick and easy meals and if desired everyone in the family can choose his or her favorite meal. Bon appetit!

Unfortunately, these new "Frankenfoods" are as guilty as Twinkies and Coke. When we became a nation of chemical eaters and foods stripped of nutrients and vitamins for the sake of color appeal and convenience a sad situation was initiated the firm evidence of which is now as easy to see as walking down the street or through a mall.

If you could step back far enough to the observe what Mrs. Cleaver and Donna Reed fed their growing families and contrast that type of food with so-called "foods" on today's market shelves you would know what happened. I sympathize with today's homemakers and their need to save time and cut corners. They are rushed, overworked and budget-challenged and my heart goes out to them.

So when processed and prepared foods came along to meet the needs of these busy, stressed out food preparers it is understandable that many thought these timesavers were gifts from the meal gods sent to ease their problems. Imagine a package with everything inside except for maybe water, milk or a bit of meat that whips up into a meal in no time. Space saving as well since there's no longer a need for flavorings and seasonings taking up cupboard space…it's all in there.

Beware! The quick and easy food gods are really a gang of Trojan horses wherein the enemy is lurking.

Later I will tell you the fascinating history of these problem solving meals and their correlation to some really scary health outcomes you need to know about before your next foray down the aisles of your friendly supermarket. This is a story with many facets and although it may appear to be a book about the dangers of processed foods, it is not. At least not exclusively. However, my research begun to try to solve the mystery of my unwanted belly led me down many dark and dingy rabbit holes.

Once the true culprit was exposed, a lot of rubble lay on the ground that could not be ignored. What began as my own personal pursuit grew into something that needed to be shared with others.

I have been fortunate to have been able to work from my home for many years. Because I love cooking, reading cookbooks, searching out new ingredients and understanding the science of cooking I have never succumbed to the prepared food appeal.

The wider my search for a culprit became the more I began to suspect the villain was hiding in plain sight but had escaped apprehension only because he was so very well disguised. In the mystery novels I write my guilty party moves through the story appearing to be as innocent as a baby lamb. How could anyone suspect someone so obviously worthwhile and decent?

When I flushed the bad guy in this story out of the bushes, at first I refused to believe the evidence. This villain was cleverly disguised as himself but not himself. When my story is told, you may call it preposterous but it will nevertheless be very difficult for you to refute the hard evidence and the resulting conviction.

Fortunately, I had a lot of excellent help from a variety of reliable and brilliant "detectives" with far more experience and resources for apprehending bad guys than I. Thus, you the reader can easily check on my claims by reading what I read in this fascinating pursuit.

What you will inevitably ask is how could something as revered and treasured have been doing so much harm for decades and so few knew what was going on. Or did they? The very idea of accusing this villain of dirty tricks played on the American public sounds un-American.

All I can say in his defense is that it is not his fault. Please forgive me for anthropomorphizing this hero turned antihero. A fiction writer uses many ploys and this is one that seems to work for this purpose. Hold onto your hat, you are about to begin a rough ride.

A mystery shrouded in history

Let us begin sometime in the middle of the nineteen fifties. If you are too young to remember the last innocent decade as I have come to call it then suffice to say that it was a time of Sputnik, the first wide-screen movies, stereo, color television, antihistamines, Mr. Potato Head, Marilyn Monroe, James Dean and Elvis Presley and Richard Nixon's famous Checker's speech.

Some of the aforementioned may have little meaning or interest for some readers but everyone knows that the post-war years brought us the segment of our current population known to us all as the Baby Boomers.

The middle of the twentieth century was an exciting time for science. Besides giving us antihistamines, a polio vaccine, oral contraceptives and the first kidney transplant along came the pacemaker for cardiology patients that eventually led to heart transplants and other miraculous medical wonders. Ah, the wonders of science.

Science however has a dark side as well. We all know about the proliferation of ways we homo sapiens have created to wipe each other off the face of the earth. Privacy is a thing of the past since anyone can know minute details of our lives in minutes and many know how to hack into our private phone calls and emails. The price of the yin and yang of being a clever innovative species. But might science also have infiltrated the food we eat in ways that they failed to tell us about that has resulted in a pandemic of obesity and sharp rises in the incidence of diabetes, arthritis, dementia, liver disease, heart disease and other killers? Surely not you say.

Remember that it is science that gave us all those quick and easy new foods that save us time, money and patience.

The results of new medicines as well as new so-called "foods" on the population can be slow to recognize. It can take decades for something new in our water, milk, toothpaste or food to show its true self. For good as well as bad.

All one has to do to view the full impact of something that science fostered on the American public about fifty years is to look around at people carrying far too much weight to be healthy.

Take that search further and check on the statistics concerning the exponential spikes in a host of dread diseases since about the mid-fifties. It would be easy to pass of these facts, pandemic obesity and increase in incidence and severity of the diseases we have come to accept as just part of life on earth until you run into some impressive research by a handful of concerned scientists and medical professionals.

Obesity is not a choice.

Obesity is the result of either poor eating (poor as in not good choices, but also the plight of being poor and eating what one can afford) or being hoodwinked by those we trust to tell us the truth and look out for our health. At least that was what many of us were brought up to believe— there are food scientists and regulators whose responsibility it is to keep us safe from dangers in our foods.

With obesity comes diabetes, heart problems, gastrointestinal miseries and other diseases not to mention embarrassment and low self-esteem.

Point of interest. The size and shape of Americans today is vastly different from say forty or fifty years ago. Think back to what John Q. Public looked like in the fifties, sixties and seventies. Take a look at photos from back then. Obesity was rare as hen's teeth.

There are actually those who blame the genes of obese people. Some people just happen to inherit fat genes. However if obesity is in one's genes then where did all those fat genes suddenly come from beginning a couple of decades ago?

There are studies that report an awareness of the increase in obesity beginning in around the early eighties. A problem like this however begins some time before it becomes fully recognized and studied. Those "fat genes" had to develop in response to something that had changed in the American diet. Yes, we can blame fast food and the proliferation of sugary and fatty foods and snacks as well as that killer the well-loved soda that bubble for bubble is as lethal as a cocked gun. More later on what the acid content in soda does to set young people up for the misery of osteoporosis later in life. Right now, we have a target in sight.

Before we shoot the arrow let us look at something that has long grated on my mind and ask you how you feel about this matter.

Let us, for the sake of argument, suppose that my earlier accusation of the dangers of prepared "food" is correct. That leads to a question of momentous importance because it is pregnant with so much contradiction that it boggles the mind.

Okay, we have all these FDA and American Heart Association and the renowned Mayo Clinic scientists, nutritionists and doctors all working, supposedly, to protect us from harm in the things we eat and the water we drink. Correct? We know the pharmaceutical industry's motives are less than altruistic since they create a market for wanna be hypochondriacs. If a pill can fix it why pull food off the shelves. That, my dear reader is counterproductive to the market. But that is a case for another day.

If the food science nutritionists are doing their job, were doing their job forty or fifty years ago, then how come they let something like "Frankenfood" on the market?

Do not fool yourself that science just got around to understanding the dangers in fat, sugar and starches that turn to sugar in the body. This is not new news. In addition, it would be naïve to think that they did not know that the big food manufacturers very cleverly found a way to take pennies worth of ingredients (many of which had been stripped of vitamins, minerals and nutrients) add fillers, artificial flavors and chemicals and call it food. Then have the audacity to advertise it as the boon to busy homemakers. All under the watchful (?) eyes of those appointed to safeguard our foods.

So why eat something with few or no nutrients? Why allow such food impersonators on the market? Silly me, we all know why. $$$$

The truth seekers know that obesity had a jump-start when these foods came along. The statistics are there to support this case. However, therein lies a deeper mystery yet to be solved. Something hidden from view cleverly disguised and yet integral to every meal we eat, fast or otherwise that will surprise you as it did me.

Sticking to my position that prepared foods are about equivalent in vitamin, mineral and nutrition content to eating the pretty packaging that encloses them let us move on. That hardly makes a solid case, you rightly say, for either obesity or spikes in say, diabetes. No, it does not. It is simply one clue whose string we must follow to the real solution.

To solve the mystery behind the obesity plight whereby fat babies grow into fat toddlers who grow into fat youngsters, teens and finally adults (adults who are diagnosed with diabetes and other diseases) we have to look far deeper than the empty calories in fast foods and prepared foods. Not that they have not and do not continue contribute to the problem every day. They most certainly do.

We all know the body needs nutrition to thrive. We get nutrition from the foods we eat. When we eat foods that provide too much fat, sugar, salt or starch imbalance occurs. Our bodies prefer to maintain an alkaline base. Too much acid and the optimum balance is thrown off kilter. Too much alkaline foods and balance is threatened. Like Goldilocks, our bodies prefer a state that is just right. That balance results from food knowledge.

The Natural Health School/ Lesson 18
Acid/Alkaline Imbalance

Over-acidity, which can become a dangerous condition that weakens all body systems, is very common today. It gives rise to an internal environment conducive to disease, as opposed to a pH balanced environment which allows normal body function necessary for the body to resist disease. A healthy body maintains adequate alkaline reserves to meet emergency demands. When excess acids must be neutralized our alkaline reserves are depleted leaving the body in a weakened condition. A pH balanced diet, according to many experts, is a vital key to health maintenance.

The A1 route to poor health is available to us in a hundred or more different varieties and flavors on both sides of the long soda aisle. Choose your poison!

Good health is a multi-faceted equation dependent on many variables. Some we can control and some we cannot. The environment has an impact on our physical health and so does our mental health. A mind full of misery sends signals that say hop on the misery wagon and ride along. A body full of useless calories, acids, and unnecessary chemicals is asking for trouble. One of the most accurate and telling phrases ever coined is the one that stated as early as 1826 but was revived in the 1920's and then again in the sixties. "You are what you eat." Think well on that one.

If you are over sixty you can recall how people looked in your youth. There was the occasional overweight person but rarely an overweight child in your neighborhood. A kid who was pudgy might have been called "fatty" but today there are scores of unfortunate children to whom the sad tag would apply. People were slimmer back then. The evidence is in those old photos.

What happened between that time and this to change the bodies of Americans? In searching out clues to this mystery the field was found to be scattered with contradictory and misleading information. At one point it even occurred to me that those who eat food that has little or no nutritional value ought to suffer from malnutrition.

Malnutrition is the condition that occurs when your body does not get enough nutrients.

We have all seen the tragic pictures of malnourished people in countries where food is in short supply. That malnutrition results in weight loss among other tragic symptoms. And yet could obese people also be considered to be malnourished because their food consumption is nearly depleted of nourishment by the process of processing? But they carry extra weight. Malnourished people waste away they do not become overweight. Therein lies the contradiction in the argument.

Nutrients: a chemical that an organism needs to live and grow or a substance used in an organism's metabolism which must be taken in from its environment. They are used to build and repair tissues, regulate body processes and are converted to and used as energy.

Added to the list of suspects is another villain. Refined carbs (no, not carbs with good manners and a taste for classical music). Refined carbs are those that have been processed and "stripped" of their basic nutrients and vitamins. White rice, white bread, white pasta, white flour for instance.

I sit here scratching my head and wondering why any food would be so cruelly treated. Whoever came up with the bizarre idea to strip foods of their nutrients and vitamins??? The concept is mind-boggling, indeed. What reasoning might there have been for doing something counterproductive to healthy eating? Here is the obvious scenario that led to stripping foods most everyone in America eats to wipe out their basic nutrients and vitamins.

Some nutcase decided that white foods are more appealing than brown foods. Hm. Now that's a new avenue to increased profits. If nothing else those white so-called "foods" would offer additional choices. And, the way to American bellies (double entendre there!) is through glossy advertising with testimonials by fake experts and movie stars. Once the public knows that white food is special and glamorous, etc. they will rush in to pull it off the shelves. Of course, not being concerned with nutrition but only with flooding the market with a fancy new product this nutcase cared not that getting a natural food into a whole new disguise meant stripping away all that is vital to food in the way of vitamins and nutrients. Way to go.

Did no one along the line from manufacturer to consumer (including the government officials who ought to have taken that course in Nutrition 101) ask the question: When is food no longer food? Answer: When food no longer provides nutrients and vitamins we might just as well eat that fancy packaging, right? Duh. Why eat 'em if they do not nourish you? Food is a delivery system well evolved by Nature to work within the body to sustain life. This is so basic and so elegant that to ignore it you have to be a mean son of a gun. Or someone lacking a conscience who is out to make a whole lot of money.

Okay, the plot thickens— as do the waistlines of Americans. If indeed the markets are full of foods with lots of empty calories and little or no nutrients then do you wonder as I do why these "Frankenfoods" ever got by the folks who are supposedly looking out for the health of the nation?

If indeed the U.S. Dept. of Agriculture happened to be napping when food producers slipped these foods whose colorful packaging is far more impressive than the contents onto supermarket shelves, when they finally woke up what did they do?

Here is the answer. Nothing. Hey, it's a free country, capitalism reigns and anyone has a right to destroy the health of unsuspecting citizens if they are dumb enough to buy the products because the advertising is clever. Right? I think it might be in the Bill of Rights. Got to check on that.

So the question is, how many of the foods on grocery store shelves have little or no nutrients and vitamins? I am hyperventilating!

What if Dr. Frankenstein had turned his hand to food creation rather than a monster?

Remember when the government-issued diet mantra exploded on the scene? Good advice, right? Avoid fats and sugars and eat lots of healthy whole grains. How many times have you seen and heard that advice? Millions (maybe billions) have been spent on getting this message to the American public. New labeling forced manufacturers to invest in new packaging.

So what are those recommended healthy whole grains? In America, home to golden waves of grain the darling of the whole grains is wheat. Farming of wheat is a huge agribusiness. Wheat farmers are a mighty force in this country.

And well they should be, there is almost nothing in the supermarket beyond the aisles of fresh produce, meat and fish that does not have a whole lot or at least a modicum of wheat as an ingredient. We like the taste of wheat and it adds texture and integrity to many products. Wheat might be said to be the magic ingredient we cannot do without.

Some time when you have nothing better to do and look forward to a day of reading labels check out this fact. I think it will surprise you.

This advice from on high caused a proliferation of Heart Healthy and Heart Friendly products to appear on supermarket shelves. The dawn of a new age.

Who among us does not want to maintain a healthy heart? Who among us does not trust the well-educated and well-informed experts who disseminate such information to the American public? So began more sensible eating. The food producers cooperated by limiting those deadly villains from their foods, sugars and fats.

Cereals and breads sporting bright red hearts jumped on the bandwagon. Even chips, cookies and crackers got a makeover to comply. Hoorah, here's to better heart health.

In the eighties we became very conscious of the information in ads, magazine articles and television food shows about carbohydrates, calories and cholesterol.

Carbohydrates n. Any of a large group of organic compounds occurring in foods and living tissues and including sugars, starch and cellulose.

Calorie n. A unit of heat energy. Calories are a measure of energy.

We need a certain level of caloric intake to keep on going. Think wood on the fire or oil in the heater. Calories over the level of basic life sustenance however turn to fat. Our bodies know how many calories we each need to sustain life and having nothing useful to do with the extras they store them as fat. Ta da!

Calories with no useful nutrients are called empty calories. Empty of usefulness to the functioning of the body. That is where sugar and fat come in. Solid fats and/or added sugar are perfect examples of empty calories. The problem about empty calories is that they add fat and that is all.

From the U.S. Dept. of Agriculture
What are Empty Calories?

Currently, many of the foods and beverages Americans eat and drink contain empty calories – calories from solid fats and/or added sugars. Solid fats and added sugars add calories to the food but few or no nutrients. For this reason, the calories from solid fats and added sugars in a food are often called empty calories.

In the book that inspired me to investigate this tangled mystery, Wheat Belly: Lose the Wheat, Lose the Wheat Belly by William Davis, M.D. a renowned cardiologist he writes about the hot catch term cholesterol.

He explains that this term is a misnomer for the reasons that it became a catch word in medicine before further studies broke down this phenomenon into its constituent parts. We also have the term "LDL cholesterol." LDL "particles" come in two sizes large and small.

"Small LDL particles are...an exceptionally common cause of heart attacks, angioplasty, stents and bypass..."

He goes on to say, "The drug industry has found it convenient and profitable to classify this phenomenon in the much easier-to-explain category of high cholesterol but cholesterol has very little to do with atherosclerosis..."

Here is where my attention really got focused in the search for verification that the villain I suspected was lurking in the lilac bushes deserved my efforts to flush him out and bring him to justice.

Those heroes of the Government's new mantra for achieving a healthier citizenry, whole grains might just not be such All-American champions after all.

Get ready for a roller coaster ride with a hard ending.

The body's processes are nothing if not fascinating. Silently, and we hope efficiently, our organs, blood, tissue and all the wondrous things that make us living breathing humans perform their magic 24/7.

They are truly perpetual motion machines. They are recyclers. They are constantly recognizing the difference between proteins, acids, sugars, starches and fats among other things like medications. But overload the well-functioning set-up by shoveling down useless junk and you will eventually know how your body feels about the situation. It expresses itself in dis-ease. From Middle English, lack of ease, abnormal and corrupt.

Is that what you want your body to report to you in no uncertain terms? I think not.

We must have become wiser shoppers since the laws that made it possible for us to read and know just what is in our food. A well-informed shopper is a prudent shopper. It would seem so but watch out for the tricksters. Those unpronounceable chemicals are one stumbling block if you do not have a degree in chemistry. In addition, those clever "food" producers have adopted nicknames for some things we have been warned to avoid.

The accepted wisdom appears to be that we should have faith in our government agencies, like the FDA and the Dept. of Agriculture to be doing the very best for us all. Faith might be fine in religion although even there is a dangerous characteristic but faith in our food purveyors may have steered us onto a very risky and slippery slope.

When science threatens to shake faith there are those who choose to deny the science and go with the blind faith. I would highly recommend that in this instance you choose the correct path. Although I will be providing lots of contradictory claims and promises, I hope that the caliber of the experts on the side of solving this mystery will convince you of existence of a nasty villain in our midst cleverly disguised as Super Man, hero to the world.

It will upset some by my saying that perhaps, there are those trusted officials who have been keeping a little secret up under their lab coat sleeves and/or designer shirt cuffs? No, no, that's incorrect. It is not a little secret but a biggie. It is enormous, gargantuan, mammoth and titanic and you and I and everyone who eats food from the grocery store deserves a heads up on this one. You can stop reading here if you grow and raise all your own food.

Okay, I have been haranguing on about my fat belly, obesity, fake foods, lost nutrients, empty calories snoozing guard dogs and such so now it is your turn to shine.

What conclusions have you arrived at regarding the common denominator ingredient that stands out as possibly being the villain for whom we are searching? Think of what you learned in high school math. What is the common denominator of these main dish foods, snacks, cereals and desserts? Excluding soda that is full of other nasty guys that lead to their own terrible conclusions in the human body. Soda contains phosphorous and carbonic acid. This criminal team is equally guilty but they are not the guys we are pursuing at the moment. A heads up for all you soda drinkers out there and that includes fans of diet soda that you erroneously believe is just fine.

Deadly Soda Drinks

FYI From Dr. Jay Adlersburg

Years of drinking too many sodas and taking in too much phosphorus can reduce bone calcium, which is a risk factor for osteoporosis. The darker the soda, such as root beer and colas, the more the phosphorus. It's one culprit.

Its not just the phosphorus in soda that is harmful. The little bubbles in soda are carbon dioxide. When they dissolve in water, they make carbonic acid.

From Dr. Wissner Greene

By the mid-thirties, bones have stopped building up appreciably, so (young) people are losing their valuable time building up bones when they drink a lot of cola beverages.

Let us set up a court-type situation now that we have all the snarky smirking bad guys in the line-up. Sugar, fat, starch, empty calories, calories in general, carbohydrates, refined carbs, low or no nutrient processed foods, cholesterol and acid/alkaline balance. Did we fail to pull in anyone else? Just to be sure the savvy attorneys dug deeper.

What they found will scare the daylights out of you and shake your faith in a number of ways.

A plethora of ailments in a loaf of bread

Closing in on the ringleader of the gang causing the serious problems facing Americans today as they struggle against unwanted pounds and strive for good health is an emotionally painful experience. The closer you get the more it appears that a lifelong friend has betrayed you.

24

One day that good old reliable pal who'd always been there with you through the good and bad times, comforting you in the low periods and sharing the highs was suddenly unmasked. There before you was not your chum but something that looked exactly like that friend and yet was not.

It was as if Dr. Frankenstein had duplicated your lifelong companion in almost every way but its essential nature. For science fiction buffs, compare the unmasked version to an android. Seemingly exact however you suspect at your gut level that your pal is missing and an enemy awaits ready to pounce.

Yes, the common denominator in all of your favorite foods is wheat. The all-American wheat. Golden waves of grain on the western plains. The staff of life. I know, I know, it would seem to be not possible and yet it is. Indicting wheat is like calling Uncle Sam a fraud. Yes, Virginia, there is a Santa Claus but Uncle Sam is an imposter.

From bread to crackers, cookies, cakes, donuts, pizza and chips wheat has a starring role. But not to be outdone wheat also takes roles ranging from bit parts to supporting actor to stooge to stage manager. Appearing in nearly every food group excluding fresh produce, meat and fish in its natural state, wheat is there doing its part to appeal to the taste of the American public. It adds texture and appeal to far more prepared and processed foods than you can shake a spoon at.

But this wheat is not the wheat my mother and aunt whipped into flaky pie crust and crunchy bread sticks. No, this wheat, wait for it…is an imposter. This wheat changed sides in the mid-twentieth century from hero to anti-hero. This wheat that we as innocent shoppers have continued to pledge allegiance to believing that it was still the staff of life went through a change at its very heart and soul decades ago and we were never warned

It was transformed from its status as all-American friend to an enemy who brought about a plague of obesity, increased incidence of diabetes, arthritis, dementia, heart disease, inflammation and gastrointestinal agony just to name a few of its crimes. And yet it roams neighborhoods hoodwinking people. Solidly backed by powerful "authorities" and "nutritional experts" who tell the American people to cut back on fats and sugars and **EAT MORE HEALTHY WHOLE GRAINS** it continues to spread its curse upon the land.

My mother and my aunt owned and ran a guesthouse on Cape Cod where I and my three younger siblings grew up. They were both terrific bread makers. Not only bread but muffins, pies, cookies, cakes, brownies and delightful fruit turnovers and bread pudding to die for (pun definitely intended). The guests raved about the wheat foods coming out of that old kitchen once habituated by a Cape Cod sea captain and his family. But back then, we were on the cusp of a new world. From a world in which wheat was the grain of choice and a trusted friend we slipped unknowingly into a whole new era.

It takes a long time, sometimes decades, for such insidious changes as obesity and the exponential rise of killer diseases to show themselves on graphs. Unfortunately, it is only in hindsight that science can view trends such as what occurred after wheat was transformed heart, soul and chromosomes from what it had been for millions of years.

This new wheat is called semi-dwarf because of its shorter stalks and larger, more productive seed heads. It has more resilient qualities to resist disease, drought, heat, etc. than the old traditional wheat. Dr. Norman Borlaug a renowned geneticist who was given the Nobel Peace Prize for his creation of this new wheat, changed the genetic makeup of the plant by around 1%. Hey, you say, that's insignificant, so what's the big deal?

That may not seem like a lot, but a similar distance stands between humans and chimps. Sometimes, 1% is a "giant leap for mankind."

By the way, Dr. Borlaug is often referred to as the Father of the Green Revolution. Green as in better food through modern chemistry or green as in big bucks for agribusiness?

The controversy over whether we are actually eating genetically modified wheat or not rages and yet, the more you read the more you wonder how the naysayers can live with themselves. Consider this: Monsanto and others say that there is "no genetically engineered wheat grown anywhere in the world today." The University of Kansas, a leader in medical and bio-chemical education sees it differently however (more on this study later). Here's the rub. Terminology. Some say hybridization and some say genetically modified (or engineered). You say tomahto and I say tomato.

In case you are not familiar with the new era of GMOs, here is a quick lesson.

Keep in mind that 1% is not to be scoffed at and set aside as unimportant. If I added 1% to the end of your nose you'd be really pissed.

A genetically modified organism (GMO) or genetically engineered organism (GEO) is an organism whose genetic material has been altered using genetic engineering techniques. These techniques, generally known as recombinant DNA technology, use DNA molecules from different sources, which are combined into one molecule to create a new set of genes. This DNA is then transferred into an organism, giving it modified, or "novel" genes. Transgenic organisms, a subset of GMOs, are organisms that have inserted DNA from a different species. GMOs are the constituents of genetically engineered foods.

It is as if your DNA was altered so that the outcome was that you grew an extra head, and one leg grew suddenly longer than the other. Now transpose that idea to a carrot. The humble carrot is engineered to have a new set of genes built into it that makes it very much not the carrot it used to be. For instance, this carrot could be not only lacking in nutritional value and have few beneficial vitamins, but it also might be dangerous to eat. For one reason, this genetic engineering often produces brand new genes (unrecognizable even to the scientists doing the work), a kind of mysterious X factor that no one should eat.

Please read twice. Sure it is technical boring stuff that to us non-scientists may sound like gobbledygook, but I would ask you to feel the essence of it. Do you feel the soul of Dr. Frankenstein in the description of what scientists might have done to your good old pal wheat?

Dr. Mark Hyman has this to say about the new wheat.

This is not the wheat your great-grandmother used to bake her bread. It is Frankenwheat–a scientifically engineered "food product" as opposed to real food, developed in the last 50 years that contains Super Gluten. This new modern wheat may look like wheat, but it is different in three important ways that all drive obesity, diabetes, heart disease, cancer, dementia and more.

It contains a Super Starch–amylopectin-A that is super fattening.

It contains Super Gluten that is super-inflammatory.

It contains something that constitutes a Super Drug that is super-addictive and makes you crave and eat more. The Bible says, "Give us this day our daily bread". Eating bread is nearly a religious commandment. But the Einkorn, heirloom, Biblical wheat of our ancestors is something modern humans never eat.

Instead, we eat dwarf wheat, the product of genetic manipulation and hybridization that created short, stubby, hardy, high yielding wheat plants with much higher amounts of starch and gluten and many more chromosomes coding for all sorts of new odd proteins. The man who engineered this modern wheat won the Nobel Prize – it promised to feed millions of starving around the world. Well, it has, and it has made them fat and sick.

The first major difference of this dwarf wheat is that it contains very high levels of a super starch called amylopectin A. This is how we get big fluffy Wonder Bread and Cinnabons.

Here's the downside. Two slices of whole wheat bread now raise your blood sugar more than two tablespoons of table sugar.

Why would universities and doctors across America dispute the Government's position on the importance of eating more whole grains if they had not done their own research? Why would they risk their reputations with fly-by-night theories in opposition to truly reliable (?) companies like Monsanto. Hey, who do you trust?

Just as frosting on the high gluten cake try this information on for size–belly size.

GM crops are not required to go through any type of independent safety peer review to determine if they are safe for either human consumption or the environment. That would be you.

The scientists who dabble in this stuff maintain the stance that "it is still wheat" so what's the big fuss? If it is still the same old wheat then why when you walk down the street or through a mall do you see entire obese families? I ask this question of my friends and people I meet at social events. Recently I asked a slim man who told me some days he doesn't eat anything. If his scale tells him he is up a pound or two he simply stops eating until the extra weight is gone.

When I opened the subject about the plague of obesity to this healthy looking middle-aged man noting that we have all registered this sad reality in the past few years he simply passed it off as lazy people who eat too much.

Easy for him to say. And although the facts cannot be denied that those who forgo exercise and eat processed and prepared foods (those Frankenfoods created in the mid-twentieth century) are doomed to carry extra weight his answer was too much of a simplification to let lie unchallenged.

Build it and they will come. Low income people must eat too. A trip to the grocery store is disheartening when you consider the price of whole food, real food like fresh produce and lean meat and fish. Astronomical.

On the other hand there are tenfold shelves of the other stuff. The quick and easy make it from a box so-called "food" that is affordable. You be the judge and jury. If you had little money to feed your family and the great American advertising community shouted at you the wonders of these foods for busy households with their eyes on precarious budgets what would you decide? The average American adult couple in the twenty-first century with two to three children, two jobs, a mortgage, car payments and no savings shops with an eye to the best food bargains. They are exhausted at the end of each day and on weekends their duties at home are piled up waiting for attention. This couple is not on the internet researching the state of food safety in America.

They only know that the amazing food industry is looking out for them, their budgets and lack of time for meal prep. It's the American way. Every day the food industry is coming up with more and more food options in the form of packaged and frozen culinary delights. Check out the International aisle in your supermarket. A bonanza of exotic offerings from cuisines around the world.

Believe it or not, among those who do exercise and try to eat right (right being the Government guidelines to cut back on sugar and fat and eat more healthy whole grains) are still battling the bulge. Particularly since they increased their consumption of those miraculous whole grains. Folks, the facts do not lie. Back in the "old days", say up through the early part of the twentieth century, fat people were the exception wherever you looked, wherever you lived, and most of them never ran except from a mouse.

Something is hiding in plain sight. Some enemy of the American people has taken hold and despite the claims of the Government subsidized food nutrition experts and companies like Monsanto, to put it bluntly, you and I have been tragically hoodwinked.

The Neurological Impact of a Ham on Rye
(Or, wheat consumption is making you crazy!)

How many times have you heard someone say, or said yourself, I'd love to lose weight, but I am addicted to food? Contrast that with, I'd love to get clean but I am addicted to heroin (cocaine, or whatever designer drug fits)?

The food addiction confession may sound like just an excuse to anyone in control of their own eating habits. After all how easy an out it is to claim food addiction rather than take responsibility for your overeating?

On the other hand, no one doubts the sad truth of the plea of the drug addict whose life is under the control of an addictive drug. The same goes for trying to quit smoking after years of addiction. Remember when the tobacco companies finally admitted to adding addictive substances to cigarettes? Nice. Addiction is a terrible thing to suffer from and almost as difficult to accomplish as growing wings and flying to Europe on your own power.

So why not a food that operates on our brain similar to an addictive drug? Maybe that is not as outlandish as it sounds. That would explain why it is so difficult to give up those Dunkin donuts or Ding Dongs after years of your body relying on the comforting sugar lift you get from these favorite snack foods. I have never smoked so I am forever questioning my former smoking friends as to what it is about a cigarette that kept them hooked. They could only compare it to the feeling of slipping into a state of relaxation with that first puff.

One friend compared it to her chocolate fix. "One bite and the world feels and looks so much better."

How would you describe that mid-morning call to seek out a snack to boost you up until lunch time? The popular term is having a "sugar low" or for those more into medical jargon, a "hypo-glycemic" slump. I am very familiar with that sudden "need" to grab something to snack on or risk all-over weakness, grouchiness, and feeling faint. Not a nice feeling and furthermore a tax on your productivity as a worker. .

It's a roller coaster ride? You eat a good breakfast and yet around ten-thirty you experience a dip. You know how to do a pick me up so you have a snack. But is this dip a mixed message? In fact, is it even necessary? If your body sugar level is under control why should you have these spikes and slumps? You know how bad it feels to slip into one. Got to get a snack fast. Then how good it feels when the need is met and things level off again. The stretches from breakfast to lunch and then again from lunch to dinner can be hell, can't they?

So what if I told you that you could eliminate the roller coaster ride of spikes and slumps, get rid of belly fat or lots of fat, and move toward avoiding some pretty nasty diseases? Bear with me and you be the judge. Because you may not have the time to do the intensive research yourself I have done it for you. I initially did it for myself and my husband so that we could lose our "wheat bellies" but the overwhelming nature and the abundance of the facts, pro and con, sat on my conscience as heavy as a donut dipped in lead. I had to share what I'd learned through hours of delving and demanding the truth.

My college major was in psychology because I had always loved studying people. In fact, I had always been a good "reader" of people. When I went back to school later in life to study Holistic Health I reinforced my already well-established theories of the importance of the mind/body connection. In fact, I had lived by the tenets of this vital approach to life for years by the time I chose to study it far deeper so that I might guide others in the practice. As such, my brain, the control center of my entire being had proved to me that it had almost magical powers for guiding all the systems in my body toward positive maintenance.

When I tell people that I "do not do doctors" I go on to explain that if I should need stitches, for instance, I'd prefer not to do them myself with my handy sewing kit. But overall I practice safe mind/body communication. Other than the crash of my thyroid a couple of decades ago (a maternal line female seemingly genetic occurrence experienced by my mother and all four of her sisters) I have been quite successful. I have been fortunate in having married a man who has contributed to the abundance of love and happiness in my life way beyond my expectations. Happiness sprinkled with lots of laughter is the best medicine by far and far less costly than illness. And yet, even though we eat only real food and walk a couple of miles a day we were carrying around unwanted frontal pouches. Thus began one of the most enlightening endeavors I have ever undertaken.

And we are now pouch-free, craving-free and for me rescued from those pesky sugar slumps. How often has my husband turned to me and said, "You need to eat, right now," when he noticed my Dr. Jekyll/Mr. Hyde slide into weakness and grouchiness? Too often. We noticed this in our darling granddaughter who would suddenly morph from charming and delightful to not so much. A quick snack returned our darling sprite to us.

I hope this book and another book I wholeheartedly recommend that you read as well Wheat Belly…Lose the Wheat by William Davis, M.D. will transform your life as it has ours and I would love to hear about your results. Be patient, believe and trust your best instincts. Something so valuable deserves some struggle to accomplish.

A mini-history lesson as a foundation for your new healthy lifestyle

The first wheat planted by the first people to take up agriculture was called einkorn and it would never pass our test for flakiness and elasticity. It produced a coarse loaf of bread indeed. Hearty and nourishing but hardly light and flaky. But to the first people to give up the wandering hunter/gatherer lifestyle and settle down on farms and in villages with reliable food sources it was a boon indeed.

Thus, began homo-sapiens' reliance on this amazing crop that supplied porridge, bread, and multitudinous wheat-based foods throughout the centuries. When wheat crops fail due to drought, floods, or disease people die, sometimes in the millions. Wars have been fought and regimes toppled because of wheat, or lack thereof.

If Marie Antoinette had not been such a ditz she would have known that if there is no flour for bread there certainly is none for cake.

Time marches on and the American public (for these purposes I am sticking to the American story but of course the story is worldwide and deeply "ingrained") develops a taste for flaky pastry, elastic pizza, scrumptious pastas, light crusty baguettes and flaky pie crusts. What the public wants the food producers supply. Or perhaps the food producers plant the idea that the public ought to want these new products. I suppose it goes both ways, to be fair to all.

The magic factor that adds the desired flakiness or elasticity to modern bread, pastries, pizza and donuts is gluten. Bakers and the public love flakiness in their wheat-based foods. The old-fashioned wheat would not do for these new demands. So science got to work and changed that old-fashioned wheat into a new modern marvel and everyone was happy.

Actually, the improvement of wheat is not a new thing in this century. No, over the millennia farmers learned how to crossbreed and hybridize to improve crops. But these processes did not affect the essential nature of wheat. Shall we call it the essence or soul of wheat? Imagine a handsome house cat in perfect health. Great coat, pointy ears, long whiskers, a cute pink nose and handsome paws (I have a weakness for kitty paws, so cute!). One day a clever scientist takes poor Fluffy into the lab and injects new genes and chromosomes into its blood stream. Fluffy goes into a cage where he is watched and monitored. Nothing much happens until Fluffy produces four adorable kittens.

In fact, they look a lot like Fluffy except for the fact that they are much smaller than Mom cat was at birth. In fact, as they grow they remain smaller overall than their blood relatives. In addition, they develop nasty dispositions and assorted unpleasant characteristics.

I prefer, as a cat lover not to follow any further on this example of genetic manipulation. Suffice to say that messing around in Mother Nature's beautifully organized and functioning gene pool is nasty business. It is one thing to breed a ginger cat with a tiger and get a handsome calico but to actually engineer the gene pool, add or subtract chromosomes (sometimes resulting in the appearance of "funky" unidentifiable new chromosomes that simply appear seemingly out of nowhere) that is really a sneaky underhanded business. And, sticking for a moment to the cat analogy, if the breeders sent these "altered" cats out to homes to befriend little children and they bit off their noses, nipped off their toes and other terrible things without warning of possible odd characteristics...

Well, it seems that is what happened when the famous Dr. Norman Borlaug began his work to improve wheat and eventually presented farmers with his semi-dwarf variety. Remember how I talked about farmers' cross-pollination of wheat striving for better grains? Even bees and birds do unwitting cross-pollination by transferring pollens from one plant to another.

But enter onto the wheat scene the clever scientists led by geneticist genius Dr. Borlaug in the mid-twentieth century who got caught up in the power play of fooling Mother Nature, not by cross-pollination but through gene manipulation. Ask yourself if there might be a downside to fooling Mother Nature by means unprecedented in the (natural) history of wheat.

Dr. Frankenstein would admire and envy these guys. They knew then what we have only heard about recently. A new word has been added to the American lexicon, gluten. Not new to the scientist however who increased that gluten by their manipulations.

Gluten glu•ten/ˈglootn/ Noun: A substance present in cereal grains, esp. wheat, that is responsible for the elastic texture of dough. Gluten n. a mixture of two proteins present in cereal grains, especially wheat which is responsible for the elastic texture of dough.

ORIGIN-via French from Latin, literally 'glue.'

From the blog 2012 Easy Health Options by Drs. Wiley, Elias and Cutler

The future of the American brain looks murky. One in 10 children reportedly suffers Attention Deficit Hyperactivity Disorder (ADHD), and millions are taking ADHD medication. At the same time, the memories of many older Americans have started to falter as they begin to experience the mind meltdown known as dementia. The possible common factor that may be driving a portion of this collective brain dysfunction: our boundless appetite for bread and other gluten-containing foods.

In other words, after you eat a meal containing gluten, your immune system may begin to attack nerve and brain tissue without an observable reaction in the walls of the digestive tract (of non-Celiac disease patients).

In fact, according to Dr. Davis, there is evidence from studying ancient bones that wheat may always have been bad for homo sapiens going back to the first cultivation of this panacea against starvation. If this turns out to be true the fact still remains that the wheat folks ate up until

Dr. Borlaug and his team did their messing with it would appear to be not as harmful as the latter day wheat.

Remember when filter cigarettes promised to cut down on the tar and such in those death sticks? Now it turns out that the effects on the smoker of filtered cigarettes as compared to non-filtered, was minimal. Just more of that billion dollar marketing hype to get Americans to subscribe to the suicide in installments plan. Smokers actually believed they could smoke more filtered time bombs than the "more dangerous" non-filtered ones. Sometimes, the level of rational thinking among homo-sapiens leaves a lot to be desired. On the other hand when the slick marketers of addictive substances lure unsuspecting customers knowing that we humans are curious critters, and they outright lie to us, well, we have to cut ourselves some slack, I suppose.

The cigarette manufacturers deserve the Fickle Finger of Fate and Blatant Nastiness award for their oh, so, clever manipulation of human brains and their addictive propensities to make multi-billions of dollars. Talk about a green revolution. The greening of America has a dark side to the one environmentalists are working to spread at a time when our planet is moaning in pain as its light is threatened with extinguishment by the alleged highest intelligent life form. You know, us with the cerebral cortexes.

What if wheat is just another addictive drug foisted upon us for the greening of corporate and agribusiness America? Chew on that elastic, flaky bit of dubious pastry.

The archeological fossil record beginning with the "new" agrarian diet (the beginning of agriculture) that included in large part the consumption of wheat shows a decline in the general health and vitality of people who switched from the nomadic hunter/gatherer mode of life to the agrarian mode. Once they settled down and began growing their own food in controlled situations there was evidence of tooth decay and degenerative diseases not present in pre-agricultural societies.

No food is perfect and no study of peoples and their diets and diseases can be complete without a lot of cross-study of environmental and social impact. However, even if we accept that wheat has never been the perfect food it has been touted to be, still it was better a few decades ago than it is now.

Here's why. Changes made at the most basic level in the mid-twentieth century by a science newly empowered with amazing insights into adding, subtracting and rearranging genes (fooling Mother Nature), give every indication of having led to the obesity plague as well as a far higher incidence of diabetes, heart disease, and gastrointestinal ailments including irritable bowel syndrome and other disturbances to good health.

When was the last time you made a cake and instead of adding baking soda you decided to opt for an equal amount of grits. Then, rather than milk you chose beer for the liquid ingredient. Then, just for fun you added some hot peppers to the mix rather than chocolate. The result would be far from the delectable birthday cake expected by your four year old. The original recipe would have yielded a far more appetizing birthday cake. Once you mess with the original formula (Mother Nature does that really well on her own) the outcome has ramifications too ugly to contemplate.

Something very important to keep in mind is that the timing of the exponential rise in weight in people in this country and the spikes in certain diseases particularly diabetes but also other autoimmune diseases have all taken place within the same historical time frame. Just a fluke or worth a closer scrutiny?

Note: An autoimmune disease is the body's improper response to its own systems, mistaking them for pathogens and thus, attacking and destroying healthy body tissue.

As scientists became better and better at altering the chromosomes and genes of crops, wheat was a perfect candidate for this manipulation. But corn and others plants got similar treatments that were considered successful. Successful for whom?

No one can argue with the question of need of healthy foodstuffs around the world and most particularly in third world countries. The improvement and increase in wheat crops is not in question here − at least not as a concept. I know, no one can eat a concept however there is much yet to learn before you come to any firm conclusions.

Like an onion, this entire wheat question has many layers and every time you remove one thinking it is the last one another is revealed.

You will be interested in this from PreventDisease.com.

The future of wheat is certain, and it's toxic. There are as many health risks associated with the consumption of wheat as there are nutritional benefits claimed by the wheat industry. Why is there such a strong emphasis on the development of wheat products all over the world when there are so many adverse and crippling effects such as neurological impairment, dementia, heart disease, cataracts, diabetes, arthritis and visceral fat accumulation, not to mention the full range of intolerances and bloating now experienced by millions of people? At some point in our history, this ancient grain was nutritious in some respects, however modern wheat really isn't wheat at all. Once agribusiness took over to develop a higher-yielding crop, wheat became hybridized to such an extent that it has been completely transformed from it's prehistorical genetic configuration. All nutrient content of modern wheat depreciated more than 30% in its natural unrefined state compared to its ancestral genetic line. The balance and ratio that mother nature created for wheat was also modified and human digestion and physiology could simply could not adapt quick enough to the changes.

The information is just as available to me and you as it is to those we trust to look out for our good health. However, if your trust level is faltering, welcome to the club.

Since wheat went through its secretive Dr. Jekyll/Mr.Hyde genetic transformation and the Government nutrition gurus jumped on the bandwagon to tell us to eat more healthy whole grains some insidious things have become apparent.

Even those respected organizations that ought to be looking out for us obviously refuse to remove the blinders, still flaunting the "party line" they encourage us to support the wheat industry. The following is a direct quote from the AARP Bulletin for July/Aug. 2112 article entitled Battling the Belly Fat.

"It's the prudent diet (that gets rid of the belly fat). It's more vegetables, more fruits, more whole grains."

Is it purely coincidental that obesity and diabetes among other dread diseases escalated in the very same time period in which wheat was going through some serious changes in its basic character?

Stretching to see the whole picture we cannot deny that this was a busy time in human history's relationship to both food and health.

Simultaneously, the records show the rise in fast food and prepared foods. Donuts and flaky pastry flooded onto the scene once the gluten in wheat was modified to make flours much more appropriate to the public's demand for lighter in composition treats. No one wants to eat a lead heavy donut or bite into a Napoleon only to find it stiff as an old shoe sole.

In addition, exercise became far more than a Sunday stroll with the family. Everyone began to exercise. Exercise clothing and gyms sprouted like weeds in springtime. Also, the pharmaceutical industry grew ten-fold. They convinced us that there was a pill, or three, for every ailment known to mankind. "Ask your Doctor if blah, blah is right for you." Who doesn't know that one? How many hypochondriacs have those scary ads produced? I know a few.

In fact, according to a number of sources but particularly Dr. Davis who takes serious issue with the pharmaceutical companies and their proliferation of pills for everything from heartburn to the agony of square toes think about this one.

Think of all the simple, natural remedies that have probably made it into the trash barrel of history because they did not lead to the release of a new pill. So, here is the dubious science in a nutshell. Better to create a pill to combat a disease or ailment even if it has been proved that removing a certain food would result in the same outcome. I know, I know, this is the ultimate craziness. Allow the suffering patient to continue consuming the guilty food while taking the pill to ease the symptoms. Whew! Does that sound to you like smoking the latest low tar cigarette as a cure for smoking. What it guarantees is that the provider of said cure will not lose business. Removing a dangerous food is a zero factor on the books. Makes you wonder if it is sensible to trust others to keep you healthy and advise you properly. Eh?

Maybe you heard as a kid what I did from an aunt who was always busy, "An idle mind is the Devil's workshop."

Maybe we need to update that saying to a body full of sugar, fats and whole grains is the Devil's workshop.

This chapter began with the problem of food addition. Is it real or imagined, you might ask. I truly love my brain so what I discovered about the effects of the increased gluten in the "new" wheat really magnetized me even more than the prospect of ridding myself of my pesky belly and once again wearing my size ten jeans.

Praise and Protect your Purkinjes

In humans, Purkinje cells (neurons located in the cerebellar cortex) are essential to the motor functions of the body and are affected by both genetic and acquired disorders. Autoimmune diseases, genetic mutations, autism and neurodegenerative diseases all are traced to the behavior of these cells. Purkinje cells have been also cited in Alzheimer's disease.

Big words that are big trouble.

Dr. Davis states in his wheat belly book that the "gluten-brain connection underlying neurological impairment was suspected as long ago as 1966..."

From a site called, Its Not Mental this: In research dating back decades, time and again, gluten has been implicated in a subset of cases that had been labeled "mental illness," including cases of autism and psychotic disorders such as schizophrenia.

A group of Scandinavian researchers even suggests that partial or complete symptom alleviation in a subset of patients labeled "schizophrenic" can be achieved with the simple solution of withdrawal from gluten.

Dr. Davis relates in his book that brain tissue such as the Purkinje cells "do not have the capacity to regenerate." Once they have been damaged it is sayonara to them..."gone forever." They are some of the largest neurons in the human brain and are solely responsible for all motor coordination. When you find yourself losing your balance on a regular basis or having difficulty walking, except for possibly knee or hip problems, the real problem could reside in these dead and dying Purkinje brain cells. According to Dr. Davis, "the antigliadin antibodies triggered by gluten can bind to Purkinje cells..." Remember the archaic Latin meaning of gluten, "glue?" Interesting? Maybe.

Wheat, among all the foods we ingest, according to Dr. Davis and others, has a special talent for producing "curious effects" in and on our brains. These effects are shared with those of opiate drugs. Save your money, beat out the drug dealers, just eat wheat!

Dr. Davis cites as examples of proof that wheat has a mind-altering effect on your brain the improvement in mood, the lessening of mood swings, improved concentration and better sleeping within just a few weeks of going gluten free. I agree wholeheartedly. So far, this paradigm change is right on for me. Better than any of those expensive and risky pills, thank you very much.

Consider this, if the gluten content in the "new" wheat is higher than in old-fashioned wheat and it has altered genes and chromosomes (according to Dr. Davis some of those chromosomes are rogues that spontaneously appeared in the mix and are unidentifiable!) should it still be called wheat?

This from a blog by David Kirkpatrick a dedicated technology watcher.

The grain we eat today has been cross-bred and hybridized so many times that its molecular structure is nothing like its original form; it's got twice as many chromosomes as it had before.

Consider what you might look like, and feel like, if the well balanced genetic formula that is you, with the right number of chromosomes to make you who you are were to be altered and the number of your chromosomes increased by a factor of two. Can you say monster?

The initial reason the first hybrids were engineered back in the early 70's was a good one – to increase crop yield and decrease world hunger. In fact, American, Norman Borlaug, was awarded the Nobel prize in 1970 in recognition of his contributions to world peace through increasing food supply. The problem is that the GMO wheat of today has never really been tested for its effect on human consumption. Yes, you read it here. No one would deny that the world needs more food, and bringing more and better food to millions is a noble endeavor. However, wouldn't you just naturally expect that the new "super-wheat" meant to solve the problem of hunger would be tested first to see if it was safe to feed to the millions? Duh.

So essentially, we have been the guinea pigs – and now we see an obese, diabetic and arthritic population in the wake of the new wheat.

The wheat our ancestors ate is not the wheat that feeds our nation today. This Frankenwheat is our enemy within. So, reflecting back on those people who are convinced that they are addicted to food (nearly all of that food that controls their eating habits contains wheat) we begin to understand the veracity of their viewpoint.

It is the sugar in foods that cause the spikes that drive us to want more. A great marketing tool, eh? When the body's sugar dives the body begs for a replacement. The cycle is on-going just like drug addiction. Compare this to the addictive additives in cigarettes.

Web site of Dr. Briffa:

…wheat-based foods are very disruptive to blood sugar (they have high glycemic index), particularly when eaten in quantity (meaning they have high glycemic load too). As a result, the pancreas will generally need to pump out plenty of insulin.

According to Dr. Davis something called polypeptides have a peculiar talent for penetrating the blood-brain barrier. The blood-brain barrier does a very effective and necessary job by protecting the brain from many substances that get into the blood that could have an adverse effect(s) on the brain. My very favorite organ (muscle?).

However, some things make it by this barrier effectively. Opiate drugs, for instance. Gluten's polypeptides have the ability to bind (glue themselves) to the brain's morphine receptor—the same receptor to which opiate drugs also bind.

I for one do not like the image of these gluten created monsters binding to my brain in the same way that say cocaine or morphine does. Is it any wonder then that people are convinced that they cannot lose weight because they are addicted to food! They are addicted!!!

What else is addiction but subservience to a substance or action (like a tic) or a food that has a firm grip on your brain? It pulls you back to it time after time regardless of your best efforts to kick the habit. Think cocaine, morphine, LSD, ecstasy and Gluten.

Dr. Christine Zioudrou at the National Institute of Health subjected gluten to some tests on lab rats to see what happens after wheat polypeptides reach the stomach. Her conclusions led to a new term in the scientific lexicon. That term is "exorphins". Or, morphine-like exogenous (having an external cause) compounds.

Compare to Endorphins.

Endorphins: n. any of a group of hormones secreted within the brain and nervous system and having a number of physiological functions. They are peptides which activate the body's opiate receptors, causing an analgesic effect.

You know, those good feelings a runner gets with the so-called "runner's high" or the feelings we get from passion. Good passion like lovemaking. You can thank endorphins for that.

However, these endogenous (internally caused) responses are built-in whereas gluten's exogeneous responses are self-inflicted. Like drinking alcohol or taking recreational or even medicinal drugs to the point of losing control of your life, gluten does some things mighty similar in your precious brain. That ham on rye could be your noon fix. The bagel at breakfast was your morning fix and unless you are a really good doobie and never give in to urges even when feeling sluggish mid-morning, you probably had a pick me up snack. In between meals fixes that come in an amazing array of choices. Dinner started with a relaxing drink and a couple of crackers and cheese. That was followed by breaded fish, a baked potato, a salad crunchy with garlic croutons and those great crusty French rolls you recently discovered at the bakery. Hey, why not just a slim slice of the apple pie leftover from Sunday dinner. The crust came out so flaky. Does the label "cuisine druggie" fit? I know this is harsh but if indeed those gluten sugar spikes are responsible, as you can be sure they are, then you can shift the blame to the national mantra— EAT MORE HEALTHY WHOLE GRAINS.

Let's suppose that tomorrow night when you sit down to watch the History Channel's special on the Civil War a flash commercial appears on the television screen. Great graphics, lots of color and a well-known celebrity in a modulated voice announces the latest from the American Heart Association. DO MORE RECREATIONAL DRUGS FOR OPTIMUM MENTAL AND PHYSICAL HEALTH. Would you?

How much wheat do you consume in an average day? How often do you experience a sugar slump? How many snacks do you crave? How many dangerous drugs do you rely on in your daily intake of food, etc.?

Here I directly quote Dr. Davis. "Wheat, in fact, nearly stands alone as a food with potent central nervous system effects."

Wheat? The staff of life ought to be as benign as good clean safe to drink water. Hm, another thought provoking conundrum.

How much do you value your brain and the brains of your family members? Do you want your children to do well in the world? Of course you do. So, what can you do right now, today, at the next meal to guarantee that outcome?

I challenge you, when you have read through this book to walk to your cupboards and refrigerator and read every label for the ingredient wheat. Hey, it is even in some lipsticks.

Then, make a new shopping list. This will not be simple at first but then what great leap for mankind ever is? At least you do not have to travel to the moon for this one. I know that most of you are time and energy constricted. I know that making ends meet these days is more difficult than ever however if you follow my guidelines at the end of the book you too can make the most significant difference in your life and the lives of your family since homo-sapiens walked out of the cave and declared, let's try a new neighborhood away from those hungry saber-toothed tigers.

Let's celebrate our power over being sheep led around the barnyard by a farmer who really doesn't give a damn about anything more than fattening us up for market.

Reclaim your brains, stop eating cardboard boxes and refuse to develop diseases so that the pharmaceutical companies can benefit from your misery. Break the vicious cycle of eat wheat, get sick, fat, and/or addicted, take a pill, keep eating wheat.

We switched to pumpernickel breads years ago because it seemed like the perfect choice compared to white bread. Natural, unbleached, whole grains, just the ticket for a nice ham on rye. Rye grains, and pumpernickel in particular are in fact the grains with the highest amount of gluten. Counterintuitive as that might be.

My mother ended her days on what seemed like a planet far away in a distant galaxy. The planet Alzheimer's. In the end, she did not recognize her four children or grandchildren and barely knew if she was alive or dead. So did my husband's mother.

If giving up wheat does nothing else but help me prevent our flying off to that distant planet then I will be delighted.

The further and deeper my research went the more I wished someone had told me this stuff decades ago.

However, the U.S. laws regarding genetic engineering supplied a neat loophole for the science. No labeling was required to let us know that a product had been "altered" from Mother Nature's original version (cross-breeding and hybridization although a kind of manipulation are however nowhere near what happens when genes and chromosomes are manipulated, added, subtracted and open to anomalies). Do not let anyone tell you that what farmers have been doing for eons is the same as what happens in the labs of America under the guidance of geneticists!

If in fact it is true (my research indicates this to be a fact) that no tests were ever conducted on humans to study the reactions to this "new" alien Frankenwheat then we have indeed been both hoodwinked and set up for trouble. When those clever food producers in the middle of the last century introduced the new time-saver Frankenfoods to the American public it was done so in a wild fanfare worthy of a hero come to save the world from drudgery and boredom. The promises of this new easy "food" made you wonder how you ever lived without packaged and prepared foods. Full of the goodness of such things as snow white rice (stripped of all nutrition and vitamins) and MSG, fake meats made from talented wheat and corn, fillers, unpronounceable chemicals and a host of imitators of real food. Hoorah!

Welcome to our shared Orwellian nightmare.

The Effect of Gamma Rays on Man in the Moon Marigolds

In the 1964 hit play and later movie, The Effect of Gamma Rays on Man in the Moon Marigolds, Tillie Hunsdorfer prepares to compete in the school science fair with her experiment involving marigolds raised from seeds exposed to radioactivity. This amidst severe family dysfunction.

Contrast the following to such a wildly far-fetched plot.

Semi-dwarf wheat cannot be grown without fertilizer, specific fertilizer, thus the fertilizer business becomes a vital component of the process. A farmer can obtain the seeds and plant acres and acres but without the specific fertilizer supplied by a specific fertilizer manufacturer his crop is doomed to complete failure. The "new" wheat is as dependent on this fertilizer as we have become on wheat. Nice symmetry there, don't you agree?

This "family" is so dysfunctional they might just as well have tried treating wheat radioactively.

So dysfunctional as to outright lie about what is going on. Read the following statements and then decide who is lying and who is telling the truth. Remember that the motivation to lie often entails protecting one's own best interests.

This from the GMO [genetically modified organisms] Compass web site financially supported by the European Union.

Right now, no genetically modified wheat is being grown anywhere in the world. Plans to introduce GM wheat in North America were abandoned in 2004. Nevertheless, scientists are still exploring ways of improving wheat using genetic engineering.

In 2002, Monsanto, the world's leading agro-biotech enterprise, submitted an application to the United States and Canada for the approval of an herbicide resistant, genetically modified wheat cultivar. Two years later, Monsanto withdrew its application.

Who's lying here?

Consultative Group on International Agricultural Research

Press Release - October 29, 1995

New wheats -- About 75 percent of all spring bread wheat varieties now grown in developing countries (not counting China) are either crosses developed by the International Maize and Wheat Improvement Center (CIMMYT), or crosses developed by national agricultural research programs in developing countries, using genetic material...

Highly recommended to me as a source of vital information because of its renowned medical and bio-chemistry departments, the University of Kansas says it all in the following.

University of Kansas

Educating Health Care Professionals since 1905

Why Gluten (Wheat) May be Bad for You

Today's modern dwarf wheat has been genetically engineered and is no longer the same wheat that ancient civilizations used to eat, and is implicated as a major contributor to obesity.

Wheat, even whole wheat products, contains starches that spike blood sugar rapidly, and can thus promote diabetes as well as causing people to age faster.

Our modern strains of wheat have more proteins that cause celiac-associated problems for people, even for those who do not have celiac disease. Up to 40 percent of the population has genes that pre-dispose them to gluten sensitivity. These people are not celiac, but can still improve their health (and lose weight) by avoiding wheat. (This means that 40% of the population is better off being gluten free).

In addition, wheat breaks down into polypeptides that can cross the blood brain barrier and act like opiates in the brain, causing some people to have a wheat addiction. And even in normal people, wheat promotes an increase in gut permeability. (This is bad)

Just for levity here is a comment from the Fat Head blog by Tom Naughton following the Grain Producer's response to Dr. Davis' book.

He quotes the Grain Producers: "Omitting wheat entirely removes the essential and disease-fighting nutrients it provides, including fiber, antioxidants, iron and B vitamins."

He goes on to say (I love this): "Ahhh, that would explain why humans became extinct during the hundreds of thousands of years we didn't consume wheat. Thank goodness those friendly aliens came to earth, planted wheat fields, then resurrected human life from some DNA samples they'd kept frozen."

This from the site, Raw-Wisdom.com

Largely between 1997 and 1999, genetically modified (GM) food ingredients suddenly appeared in 2/3rds of all US processed foods. This food alteration was fueled by a single Supreme Court ruling. It allowed, for the first time, the patenting of life forms for commercialization. In just those three years, [1997-2000] as much as 1/4th of all American agricultural lands or 70-80 million acres were quickly converted to raise genetically-modified (GM) food and crops. And in the race to increase

GM crop production versus organics, the former is winning

No, this is not meant to be another conspiracy theory book. I wish it was, then I would not be so damned upset by the scary conclusions presented here.

When you consider that the authorities most Americans look to for their information on nutrition and medicine may have done them a huge wrong a few decades back they do begin to seem suspect of conspiracy. I for one must say that what I have uncovered in this investigation, the result of hundreds of hours of reading, searching and delving angers me right down to my newly gluten free bones.

For instance, just ask yourself what might those life forms be that can be patented for commercialization? Eight-foot tall four hundred pound hybrid creatures that are a cross between saber tooth tigers and nasty fishercats? Just train one to guard your front yard and frighten off burglars? The marketing potential is profound. Whatever new life forms science can create and prove to have a commercial potential are protected by a Supreme Court ruling. Does that scare you? Think about that in the middle of the night when sleep eludes you.

When the powers-that-be agreed with the geneticists who contrived semi-dwarf wheat strains that the result was "still wheat" they colluded with them against the American public. How else might I put it?

Whatever the reasons for the healthy whole grains scam, you can rise above it and refuse to be led around by agribusiness. Wheat might be the staff of life but gluten can really stick it to you. The good news is that it is not your fault that you consume this killer ingredient many times each day. Those all-knowing trusted experts on nutrition and good health led us all down the proverbial garden path with their multi-million dollar campaign designed to get Americans off high fat/high sugar diets. How do you feel about half-truths?

Misinformation disseminated from the very top of the scientific community jumped on the other end of that seesaw in the middle of the twentieth century and sent us all flying helter-skelter. The line in the sand would be obvious to anyone conscientiously making a study of the increase in population-wide body weight, the spike in diabetes, coronary health, dementia, gastrointestinal complaints, etc. since that time. Many professionals have already tabulated and recorded these upsetting facts.

More recently, the nation-wide statistics on knee and hip replacements has burgeoned. Of course, this study must take into consideration the fact that the joint replacement phenomenon exists because of this miraculous scientific breakthrough in the scientific engineering of such marvels. However, necessity being the mother of invention, perhaps the chicken and egg question rears its head on this score as well.

After all, if people's knees and hips remained vibrant and healthy naturally there would be no demand for such devices. A billion dollar devise and surgical market gone. Boo hoo.

Not that our joints do not grow old and lose their flexibility, until we conquer the problems of aging this will occur. However the #1 villain wheat has also been at work there eroding away vital cartilage and being generally nasty.

Unfortunately, it does not stop there. Those man in the moon marigolds never caught on because of the difficulty of obtaining really good gamma rays. However, if you like nice hearty flowers with large blooms and thick stems you might like the sight of your bloated internal organs on wheat.

Give my regards to your big fat internal organs

To use some popular jargon, this next information will really gross you out. It certainly did us.

Shall we begin with some terrible imagery? Why not? Foie gras, big fat juicy goose liver is expensive and highly regarded by gourmands. No fun for the goose however.

Penned up so that the possibility of any exercise is verboten, geese are force fed through tubes thrust down their throats until they nearly explode from obesity. The reason: A fat goose means a nice fat liver. A nice fat liver has a nice hefty price in the gourmet market. Foie gras, truffles and caviar are probably some of the world's most expensive delicacies.

Our livers however prefer to be comfortably small and compact with only the normal amount of fat. So it is for the kidneys, pancreas, colon and intestines. Not to mention the life pump, the heart.

The torso can be likened to a climate controlled storage facility that is home to all the vital organs except for the brain. All things being equal, the organs function at optimum.

The belly fat that Dr. Davis has dubbed "wheat belly" is also called visceral fat. That fat that settles stubbornly in the abdomen can thank its sources wheat gluten, fats and sugars. Or curse them. These same culprits, if not restrained continue to march into all the body's tissue until obesity reigns.

But here is the kicker. You cannot have a fat abdomen without nice plump organs. Think about it, that would be an impossibility. The visceral fat takes over the entire storage facility and all of its occupants. And plump organs are inefficient, hard-working, stressed and faster ageing organs that become far more susceptible to disease than normal sized organs.

So here's to your big fat liver, kidneys, pancreas, intestines, colon, etc. and the big guy—the heart. Nice imagery or scary enough to make you defy all the nice warm and fuzzy advice from the powers that be who want you to increase your daily consumption of whole grains?

Or you can choose to be foie gras on toast points.

I can tell you that as much as I was concerned about fitting into my clothes and looking down at that unwanted frontal pouch, becoming informed of my big fat organs really sent me into orbit.

Earlier I mentioned that there are stats on when people began putting on far more weight than had been the normal previous trend that has come to be referred to as the "explosion in obesity." Likewise there has been a simultaneous explosion in the incidence and intensity of diabetes.

This from Dr. William Davis' Wheat Belly book

1985 [is] the year when the Centers for Disease Control and Prevention (CDC) began tracking body weight statistics, documenting the explosion in obesity and diabetes that began that very year.

…these trends take time to gather momentum and become recognizable. By the time we were told to double up on whole grains while cutting down on sugar and fats it was becoming pretty obvious that obesity was becoming pandemic. The fact is that those grains, in various forms, with and without nutritional value and inherent vitamins were already out there doing their thing. Yes, sugars and fats had become increasingly more prevalent in foods. As the American palette became more educated and simple porridge for breakfast did not satisfy, the food producers answered the need.

Boring old porridge was replaced first by a few new and exciting cereal offerings. Then those offerings exploded to fill shelves and shelves of supermarkets with scrumptious sugary cereals made more appealing with a rainbow of artificial coloring. What is the principal ingredient in cereals? In fact, it is called a "cereal grain". You know the answer. Wheat. Combine wheat, sugar and suspect artificial coloring and you get a whole new enemy within. A three-fold sugar spike you could climb like Jack did that bean stock.

Check out packaged foods for the primary ingredient. Ditto the frozen foods and condiments and even lipstick. Lipstick?

What if obesity did not have to happen and diabetes was now relegated to the status of a defeated disease of the past like bubonic plague? What if tests on humans of the "new" wheat had shown all of the potential dangers of encouraging Americans to eat more healthy whole grains? What if pigs could fly?

Like the American flag, wheat holds a position of national pride and allegiance. And is an enormous income producer for agribusiness.

No one wants farmers to go under. No one wants people to starve. No one has an argument with making money in our commercial society. But what if the powers that be, when faced with an ugly reality took measures to prevent the potential for obesity, increased incidence in diabetes and other diseases? These diseases, do not forget, cost the sufferers (most of whom do not have health insurance) create an increased demand on medical services and ultimately weaken and kill the people of this nation. We the People.

So are we supposed to blame those talented geneticists who created semi-dwarf wheat and other manipulated foods and assumed that their end-product was still the same old healthy wheat or corn, etc.? Or do we blame the Supreme Court for opening up a Pandora's Box and releasing control over new life forms a la Dr. Frankenstein?

But why would they mess around with such a sacred cow? A term we have all come to know is agribusiness.

Agribusiness n. agriculture conducted on strictly commercial principles.

Think about that for a moment. Operative word, principles. When big money enters the picture in any enterprise do certain principles go out with the, in this case, the chaff? You bet they do. Consider the pharmaceutical industry and the wellness industry overall. Should you require medical attention the very first concern for the provider is, Can you pay? Okay, service has a price, but what if that principle was applied to every interaction you have in your daily life.

Every interaction that you have with your loved ones, friends, and co-workers demanded that you be so mercenary that every word and action was contrived to elicit a payback

66

financially? How principled would that be? Now multiply that by billions.

This from the site simply called Grain.

GRAIN is a small international non-profit organization that works to support small farmers and social movements in their struggles for community-controlled and biodiversity-based food systems

Back in the early 1990s, many of Seedling's pages were devoted to discussions about international treaties and public research agendas. Corporations were part of the discussion, but mainly as a looming threat, one group of actors pushing forward the industrial model of agriculture that was destroying agricultural biodiversity. Fast-forward twenty years, and the landscape has changed. Corporate power in the food system has grown by leaps and bounds. Today corporations set the global rules, with governments and public research centers following their lead.

The fall-out of this transformation for the planet's biodiversity, and the people who look after it, has been devastating. Corporations have used their power to expand monoculture crop production, undermine farmers' seed systems and cut into local markets. They are making it much more difficult for small farmers to stay on the land and feed their families and communities. This is why social movements are increasingly pointing to food and agribusiness corporations as the problem in the global food system and the focus of their resistance.

In case you are not familiar with the term monoculture, heads up.

Monoculture: Monoculture is the agricultural practice of producing or growing a single crop or plant species over a wide area and for a large number of consecutive years. It is widely used in modern industrial agriculture and its implementation has allowed for large harvests from minimal labor. However, this ratio remains true only if the accounting for labor required is limited to the number of workers employed on the farm. If the indirect work of employees involved in producing chemicals and machinery are taken into account, the ratio of labor to output is higher.

Monocultures can lead to the quicker spread of diseases, where a uniform crop is susceptible to a pathogen.

Which begs the question: What if this one plant species (semi-dwarf) that is favored by agribusiness and recommended to farmers struggling to hold onto the family farm had not come along to nearly wipe out bio-diversity in grain farming?

It looks as if this one plant species, the result of genetic manipulation, is guilty of shifting the axis of our diets not long ago. This plant in its new up-dated, higher chromosome count, gene-altered state (it seems) has resulted in a host of problems that might not exist if the "old-fashioned" grains that proliferated before the big guys began devouring the market and dictating the terms had been stopped in their tracks.

I happen to be a serious student of history and as such I am aware that there are things that fall under the heading of progress that smack of retrogression flashing in bright neon colors.

Progress for some is the ruin of others. Just take for instance, the so-called "progress" in the big bank oligarchy due to setting these vultures free from all controls that destroyed many lives and left millions jobless and homeless. Progress for whom?

So, suck in your wheat belly and glory in your big fat engorged, foie gras organs or pick up your fork and rebel.

Before moving on a little pep talk.

Despair not, being free of gluten does not mean being deprived of bread, cookies, crackers, chips, pie, pizza etc. Pasta too just got a break after being a culprit for so long. Cheese and eggs just received a pardon after years of striking fear in the American heart as those baddies responsible for our overweight population and the rest of us battling whatever bulge we carried around semi-acceptingly.

The skinny (pun definitely intended) on the gluten free diet, in capsulized form is this: If you do not have an allergy to dairy (and that allergy remember might not be a stand-alone but exacerbated by wheat) and all else being equal in your health you stand to win big when you go gluten free.

When I told some friends recently that there are other cooking and baking flours out there other than wheat I watched eyes glaze over. When I told them we eat our favorite blueberry pancakes, pizza, pies and brownies among other things, they looked mighty doubtful.

"But you gave up wheat so shouldn't you be following a one-dimensional boring diet just for the sake of your post-menopausal belly that every woman knows is a given at this age and must be tolerated." That from a dear friend who loves food as much as I do and who has given up fighting her belly pouch.

Then I listed coconut flour, chick pea flour, chestnut flour, almond flour and rice flour. The only reason we have been trained to believe that wheat is the only type of flour is because of the long history of that national hero wheat in our diets, and more recently, the wheat lobby.

Yes, new ingredients call for altering baking and cooking skills so deeply "ingrained" in those who still employ those old-fashioned skills. But believe me, eating real food rather than Frankenfood pays off in so many ways you will be willing to put in a bit more time. Surprisingly, there is joy in preparing real meals and they do not take much more time than those boogey man foods. Would you rather spend your time in the doctor's office or in the kitchen?

Aye, there is the rub. Going gluten free calls for a huge commitment to resist the easiest way to provide meals for your family. So far, there are gluten free packaged foods however you must also read labels for too many starches like potato starch, tapioca starch and cornstarch. Moderation. Patience, determination and moderation. Steady on sailor!

We are totally convinced with the results that are manifesting daily to our pure delight. My husband's abs look the way they did when I met him on the beach in 1982. My waistline, long missing and missed is making a comeback. When I look down, I no longer see that pouch that might have doubled for a fanny pack. Gone, gone, gone. My appetite and cravings are under control. My (our) relationship with food is quite changed. We have more energy and we sleep better.

Best of all is the loss of those big fat internal organs. I mean, the term "bighearted" has definitely taken on new meaning.

More to come. Start salivating.

Threshing for the whole truth

I am old enough to have lived through wheat's transition from the flour my mother used to make her wonderful Christmas cardamom bread, her spectacular lemon meringue pie and date turnovers of which I could eat a half dozen at a sitting. Bread and pastry were integral to my generation's sense of home and comfort and security.

My Uncle Frank Kavanagh despite advise not to because the Great Depression still held the country in its grip did start a new company Mrs. Kavanagh's English muffins in the mid-thirties. The wheat that went into those delicious muffins with the nooks and crannies where butter sat in little warm pools is as different from today's wheat as yesterday's cotton clothing is to today's polyester. One is natural and the other not. Plain and simple.

My mother and her contemporaries wore girdles and before that it was the constricting corset that interestingly enough encouraged dieting by not allowing overeating by its very nature. The fact is that these ridiculous customs for binding the middles of females were not instituted necessarily to hold in excess belly fat. Overweight people were more commonly the well-to-do, think Henry VIII and his cronies. Shakespeare's Falstaff whose apt nickname was "fat guts" was obviously getting his share of loaves from the castle kitchen. The wealthy merchants and industry leaders, the guys who lived in grand homes and ate whatever they wanted were easy to spot. They were robust with popping buttons on their vests crossed by gold watch chains. Pudgy fingers sported huge gold and diamond rings and their whiskers sprouted from pudgy jowls. The poor could be very thin but average income people in society (the middle class were pretty much trim and lean.

So the tight corsets and later Maidenform girdles were really just because the fashions of the times demanded thin, thin, thin. Fashion models were super thin in the fifties and sixties thus, every fashion conscious woman was on some kind of slimming diet in the sixties, seventies and eighties. Everything from the grapefruit diet to the African mango diet.

Wheat was also in fashion as it has been for millennia but the average person was not overweight. It does not take Sherlock Holmes and Watson to dig through the evidence for the nasty culprits.

The grain we Americans most like to eat goes through a lot of stress on the way to our tables or tailgates. We grind it, pull it, roll it, put it through compression machines (pasta makers) and all kinds of operations to make it tasty and pliable for any number of processed foods.

A processed food is any food that is "handled" a lot on the way to your table as opposed to fresh produce, meat and fish. Processed foods have additives like flavorings, MSG, preservatives, added fats, sugars, starches and dyes. Not only the principal ingredient in most packaged food is wheat but MSG is made from wheat. It is there to enhance flavor. You know, like the additives in cigarettes that cause addiction. But that is just the beginning. Processed foods are cooked, frozen, dehydrated, milled and who knows what else. Talk about manipulation.

The plain fact is that any food that is subject to various and sundry manipulations before we eat it is a bit like accepting the regurgitated food a mother robin slips down her baby's gullet. Pre-chewed or at least softened by saliva or stomach acids. Great for growing robins but our systems work quite differently.

Our digestive systems are set up to do the work of the mother robin. However, when "food" arrives already "chewed" it does some funky things in there. Pre-manipulated, starches, fats and sugars are not as easily recognized thus, the sorting and shipping department gets a bit confused

The foods we eat are sorted, packaged and shipped along to the places that require them for smooth operation. The pancreas, for instance, deals with sugars and strikes a balance by producing insulin if needed to keep things humming along nicely. It is when things go awry that the pancreas increases its output because of faulty messages in the delivery system and this can lead to diabetes.

Sugars per se are not the enemy. Sugars turn into glucose to fuel metabolic reactions in our cells. This is a good thing. Glucose is the most common sugar and an important facilitator of a properly functioning body. No, a bag of Dunkin donuts is not a health food.

But too much or too little glucose disturbs the balance. Sugar that has been processed or refined is bad for the body. In a perfect world we would all return to the Paleolithic diet but that is highly unlikely for the majority of us. However, the opposite to being a hunter/gatherer is not the frozen, prepared, processed food aisles in your supermarket. Therein there be monsters!

What I am about to tell you flies in the face of what those heart healthy and heart friendly labels appearing like dandelions in spring on everything from "whole grain" cereals, crackers, pasta and breads to processed foods want you to believe.

Processed whole grains…wait for it…turn more rapidly and dangerously into glucose than other foods. That ham on rye is more dangerous for your health than a candy bar.

So why have the so-called nutrition experts who want us (rightly) off fat and sugar consumption given us the palliative of whole grains that cause larger and higher and more dangerous sugar spikes than sugar???

Dr. Davis explains in his book that the carbohydrates in wheat are composed of repeating chains of the simple sugar glucose called polymers. Unlike the simple carbohydrates such as sucrose which are one or two unit sugar structures these polymers are repeating chains (I get an image of the familiar colorful DNA chain).

According to Dr. Davis it is because of the changes in wheat in approximately the past fifty years driven by the demand for the flaky donuts sold on nearly every street corner and light as a feather cupcakes and fancy wedding cakes that can only succeed when made with "designer" flours that our favorite grain has been turned into "Frankenwheat."

Here are some quotes from a report from the Sierra Club regarding the state of genetically engineered crops in the U. S. Wheat is not specifically named.

"…genetically engineered organisms (GEOs) are being released to the environment on a massive scale, an event unprecedented in the 3.8 billion year history of life on this planet. This technological upheaval happened virtually without public debate, while our government played the role of enthusiastic promoter, rather than cautious regulator, of this radically new and environmentally hazardous technology.

By 1999, almost 80 million acres of North American farmlands were planted with genetically engineered seed. This means massive releases of GEOs to the environment are now taking place. Genetic engineering now poses a very grave threat to the natural environment.

Over 60 percent of all processed foods purchased by U.S. consumers are manufactured with GE ingredients. Some corn and potatoes have even been genetically engineered to contain a gene from Bt bacteria which causes every cell of the plants to produce an insecticidal toxin. Yet there is no labeling of these or any GE foods as being genetically engineered, because the U.S. Food and Drug Administration (FDA) considers the GEOs from which these foods are made to be "substantially equivalent" to the non-genetically engineered plant from which the GEOs are derived.

Dr. Mark Hyman who in involved in research into the root causes of chronic illnesses has this to say about the "new" wheat.

This is not the wheat your great-grandmother used to bake her bread. It is a...scientifically engineered food product developed in the last 50 years.

Suffice to say that in the digestive tract 75% of the chain of glucose units called amylopectin and the 25% called amylose are digested by the salivary and stomach enzyme amylase. The former is efficiently digested to glucose while the latter is much less efficiently digested resulting in its making its way to the colon undigested. The amylopectin that has been converted to glucose is absorbed by the bloodstream and is responsible for wheat's "blood-sugar-increasing effect".

Other carbohydrate foods, according to Dr. Davis also contain amylopectin but not the same kind as in wheat. As Dr. Davis puts it, the most digestible form of amylopectin is the kind found in wheat. Hold onto your hat and all that you have been taught and hold dear about the goodness of wheat in the diet. Eat more whole grains????

According to studies done by Dr. Davis, wheat increases blood sugar to a greater degree than a candy bar, hot fudge sundae or a frosty glass of Coke.

Sure maybe the eat more healthy grains campaign got people to cut down on their fat consumption however did they simply swap one serious health problem for another? Filtered cigarettes for non-filtered.

The proliferation of whole grain breads cereals and pastas etc. flashing the orange or white labeling promising the product is heart healthy may have instilled an artificial confidence in the American public that is unforgivable if the facts hold up as they seem to be doing.

So if you are wondering why your blood test showed an elevated blood sugar score and your doctor used the term "pre-diabetic" maybe it is time to become a doubting Thomasina or Thomas.

My research into a number of studies into the dangers of wheat gluten indicate that hybridization and genetic engineering of wheat has resulted in a staggering 500 fold increase in the gluten content of modern day wheat. If we compare this gluten content to the wheat our ancestors grew and ate it begins to look mighty suspicious. Wheat went through a major character change in the twentieth century to meet the demand of bakers and the public.

Yes, we discerning foodies, lovers of everything about food, always open to the latest innovation and oh, so fond of flakiness in our light as air pastry and bread were the drivers of this market demand for designer flours. Or were we? Perhaps the reality is that it was six of one and half dozen of another. Around the world gourmet chefs are always anxious for the latest innovation in foods and food preparation. So it was only natural that the demand for better flours with more talents was heralded.

Thus the wheat producers listened and complied. But at what price?

Who would have guessed that refining wheat for different characteristics would be bad for the health of the world? We cannot all be trained food scientists or food science watchdogs. Thus, we put our trust in those who are. It can make your head spin to hear and read the latest food enemy and the recommended diets that jump onto the band wagon each time a food is declared bad for us.

Remember the egg scare when we all limited our egg consumption to Sunday brunch? And yet a three egg omelet triggers no spike in glucose but add a slice of whole wheat bread and blood glucose levels spike phenomenally.

Carbohydrates have rightly been identified as enemies of good health. Not carbohydrates per se because our body needs carbohydrates for energy. However, there are good carbohydrates and then there are the bad guys. From the Insulite Lab doing intensive research into female health issues.

Addiction to carbohydrates and gluten often underlies excess weight and obesity.

As many as 75% of overweight and obese people in the U.S. may be addicted through poor eating habits to either carbohydrates or the protein called gluten, which is found in all wheat, rye, barley and oat products.

Like any addiction, these cravings are unhealthy and problematic. They take the form of either an irresistible craving for carbohydrate-rich foods such as desserts, candies and junk food, or gluten products like breakfast cereals, breads and pasta. Carbohydrate addiction is, in fact, caused by excess insulin, which is released by the pancreas into the blood stream when carb-rich foods are eaten. Insulin signals the body to take in food, then, once the food is consumed, orders the resulting energy to be stored in the form of fat. Too much insulin results in an irresistible and frequent desire to eat.

A vicious formula, indeed. Gluten-Fats-Carbohydrates-Sugar=Addiction=FatOrgans=Fat Body=Increased Addiction.

Note: Even if you are slim, no belly and no cravings you still may be playing with fire by eating those so-called "healthy whole grains." As you age, your body goes through changes that wheat can adversely affect. An ounce of prevention now is worth a healthy longevity later.

My journey to a gluten free lifestyle: A personal journal of discovery

As a child I could have modeled for an art class doing drawings of stick people. My high revving metabolism was the wonder of everyone I knew. No matter what I ate or in what amounts I never put on an ounce. After my mother stopped worrying that I'd break like a small twig and turned to worrying about how she was going to keep up with my appetite, all was well.

She was a terrific baker and dessert maker. In fact, for a few years she was the pastry chef at the renowned French restaurant Chillingsworth in Brewster the town I where I grew up on Cape Cod. I and my siblings were never short of home baked bread, brownies, cookies, pies and she put crunchy homemade bread crumbs on top of my favorite meal baked macaroni and cheese. Yum.

When it was time for me to take over my own kitchen I read cookbooks in bed like novels. Gradually I learned to be a pretty good cook myself. I cite the publication of the Silver Palette cookbooks as a watershed period in my cooking. Julie Rosso and Sheila Lukins, taught me to cook far more "artistically". Food shopping and preparation became for me wonderful art forms. I am probably one of only three people in the world who love grocery shopping. I love the acquisition of food. The colors of produce delight me and sometimes I simply stand surrounded by beautiful vegetables and fruits and absorb the wonder of it all! (I am also a painter so I guess some of goes to my love of color in painting). As I go through the market I have a pretty good idea of what meals I want to make that week but also I let foods inspire me as well.

A lovely fennel bulb can reach out to me begging me to slice it thin and grille or bake it along with other root vegetables and serve it with loin pork chops topped with a basil and sun-dried tomato pesto. Before I moved from being a landlubber to living part of the year on our boat and part following the sun to Puerto Rico I always had a large garden. I cannot cook without herbs so I grew my own and still do in pots on the boat.

Good breads have always lured me. A trip to France however spoiled me forever toward American breads so I began baking my own. Life rolled on and my belly fat accumulated post-menopause and after my thyroid "went down". All the females in my mother's family, my mother and my four aunts suffered from hypothyroidism that occurred between forty and fifty. The end of my career as a world-champion eater.

Ken's tight abs began to disappear when we moved in together because as a bachelor cooking for himself he cooked simply and ate less than he did after he met me and was captured by my Food Is Love mentality.

We were not happy about these developments but since we were not fat all over we chalked it all up to ageing. Yet somehow I was not willing to accept that I had to tolerate a pouch that no matter how straight my posture and how aggressively I pulled it in the belly still sat there seeming out of character for the rest of my body. Sure, I had put on a few mid-life pounds and would never weigh in again at the size I was back when I did some professional modeling in the fifties and sixties. But, all things considered, it was only the belly fat that belied my personal pride in keeping my body in good shape.

In addition, the more I read about excess weight in middle age and the dangers of heart problems increasing with each added pound, I could not shake my concerns about our bellies. Why were we reasonably slim and yet we carried these fat sacks on our fronts? And, we were food conscious. No processed foods, lots of fresh veggies and fruit, no sugar, no soda, no fast food and yet, the belly. We faithfully followed the national campaign to reduce fats and sugar and eat more healthy whole grains. Uncle Sam said it so it must be true.

I became suspicious last year when I read an article about people who are certainly more athletic than we are with our daily walks but who still could not shake all the belly fat accumulation. Since we have become a nation of "everyday" athletes who run, fast walk and belong to gyms we ought not to have this problem. At least, those serious "everyday" athletes ought to have rid themselves of the wheat bellies.

My parents and their friends did not belong to gyms and a walk was a stroll on Sunday afternoon after dinner. There were no gyms except for the professional athletes. Something was amiss. So, when I happened upon the wheat belly book by Dr. Davis I knew I'd found the light at the end of the tunnel. What I read astonished, angered, confused, annoyed and ultimately enlightened me.

Being a person who, despite how impressed I might be with one source of information on a subject, must find supporting evidence in as many places as possible, I was off and running. I set aside a new fun mystery I am writing featuring a cat sleuth to delve for answers.

Remember how I admitted to loving grocery shopping, well, I also love doing research. In college I thrived on doing research papers. That quirk in my character (?) has however come in handy when I am writing my mysteries. My love of history and mystery combined send me on fascinating searches for obscure facts for my books.

However, I had no idea of how deep this gluten well would be when I began.

Hundreds of hours later, after digging through the miasma of contradicting information reeking with lies, innuendoes and outright evil-doing as well as good solid honest and concerned reports from good honest concerned people and institutions I want to share. No, I must share. What I have learned constitutes something way beyond what the average person suspects. And because my readers are all leading busy and demanding lives with little time to budget to similar research I hope this helps them to make wise health decisions.

I am fortunate to be a full-time researcher and writer who has the time to dig through this enormous mountain of misinformation and deceit to uncover the truth. For myself and my readers.

Dr. Davis taught me the term "visceral fat" and the light came on. When he explained how this type of fat accumulates and why our favorite grain makes us both hungry and fat I knew I had found a kindred spirit. Dr. Davis' credentials are impressive and his motivations admirable. As a cardiologist he sees "cross-over" patients. Heart problems stemming from or sharing space with other health conditions in a kind of invisible symbiosis. Over the years of his practice and because he once suffered from being overweight and conquered it he has come to conclusions about wheat in our diets that everyone should know.

My husband and I were fully convinced after we read the wheat belly book. In fact, even before I began my research for an even broader understanding for us, as it originally began, we went "cold turkey" and gluten free.

The best thing we have ever done for our general health and our mid-life shapes! As the information piled like a part dung heap and part brilliantly shiny hill of enlightening revelations boggling my mind and challenging my beliefs in a plethora of things I had once taken for granted I knew this stuff must be shared with others.

When I received an email from an old friend who read my "blog" on Facebook about my intentions to compile my research into a book, I knew I was on the right track.

This woman had been my two children's babysitter years ago. Over the years she had put on far too much extra weight and although she was sure she ate well nothing helped. Diets, exercise, whatever she tried failed. When her doctor recommended Dr. Davis' book and shortly afterwards she read my message she emailed me bubbling with delight.

Thank you Janice. I hope this helps you as well as everyone fighting the battle of the bulge. There is an enemy hidden within the American daily diet and if the powers-that-be had their way you would never be privy to its existence.

To quote Dr. Davis, "We as a well-fed, well-informed nation are in fact "hungrier and fatter than any other time in human history." See the contradiction yet?

When our doctor told us last spring (2011) that our blood sugar was very high and we were "prediabetic" our world tipped on its axis. Us, conscientious eaters like us?

And by the way, just in case you are a man worried about those developing or already developed "man boobs" this is the book for you.

This visceral belly fat produces the hormone estrogen. That can result in "man breasts" but far worse leads to other inflammatory responses that can lead to heart disease and others problems. Inflammation by the way is a key term here. Inflammation is at the source of far more medical problems than most people know. The inflammation of your big fat belly is also responsible for taking everything inside it on the same ride. So, give my regards to your big fat organs.

Or join me on a journey to a better, healthier gluten free lifestyle.

Putting it all into perspective and practice

Now we had to put into practice what we had learned. I am an all or nothing type of person who does not see the point of taking baby steps if one giant step can get you to something desirable and get on with it. In addition, I practice a lot of mind over body control. Unfortunately, when my mind was clogged with gluten there was some interference!

I firmly believe and have clearly seen the evidence that negativity in the control center filters down to the whole system. People who have nothing but defeatist thoughts usually adversely affect their general health.

Once we both became convinced that Dr. Davis knew what he was writing about and my long in-depth research further convinced us to go for the gold, we never looked back.

However, looking down after ten days to find that our frontal pouches were mostly missing sparked a real thrill of accomplishment. When an experiment based on deep commitment and belief in the process pays off and you know you are on the right path life feels really good.

Once Ken also agreed to go cold turkey, to jump in at the deep end, throw our cards on the table and, as Ken said, "…get off the loaf, the sky was the limit. It certainly helps when you have a best friend sharing the commitment, comparing results and being supportive, so try to do it with a friend.

Dr. Davis warns that going gluten free might cause some people to experience withdrawal symptoms. Addiction does that. However, it is my contention that the withdrawal symptom are more likely to be emotional rather than physical and easily overcome with the proper attitude.

Sure, in the beginning, the first time we went out to dinner at a restaurant and got a funny look from the waitperson when we said, "Please no bread and hold the breadcrumbs on the broiled haddock and the croutons on the salad," we giggled. The next time however our waitress knew about the gluten free lifestyle and we struck up a great conversation.

Dinner at a friend's house was preempted by apologizing for having become finicky eaters but explaining that it really isn't too difficult to accommodate us. Now our friends all know and beg for more information. As with all new heightened awareness one begins to notice the contradictions all around. I picked up a Diabetes Guide to Eating booklet and read the strong recommendations for eating whole grains. Wheat flour was listed in recipes for cakes and pizza.

Okay, with anything not only new on the scene but so contradictory– and, in fact, openly threatening to the wheat industry– one must expect a long period of transition to acceptance. How often do you hear of a new breakthrough in medication for something that will be a boon to Americans and then hear that it will not be available for ten years? What on earth is that all about? Are the scientists really sure of their discovery? Are the pharmaceutical people geared up to produce it? And the big question, if it is the next big solution to some terrible disease or condition how many will suffer and die before it hits the streets? I do not mean something questionable but I have heard these hopeful announcements followed by, "available in 2020. So why even tell us?

This gluten thing is big. Yes, as with any new discoveries the ramifications are enormous. Someone always loses and someone always wins. But I would like to go out on a limb and say that as your volunteer test case I truly am convinced of these results. Visceral weight loss, a big decrease in appetite alarms, the wipeout of cravings, better sleep, more energy and an all-over sense of being up-lifted.

On the visceral fat front: If you are overweight in general, not just annoyed by a pesky frontal pouch, the pouch will begin to go first and then the rest of the weight will follow.

Two stand-out things for me are certainly knowing that I am healing my engorged internal organs and my brain is regenerating and will last longer as I age. I do not want to go to that distant galaxy and the planet Alzheimer's, ever.

Having been addicted to riding the nasty roller coaster of sugar spikes and the unpleasant symptoms at the bottom of the ride when feeling weak and faint and becoming Georgina the Grouch dictated my life every few hours I am here to say, Hello, my name is Cynthia and I was a wheat addict. But no more.

You can make a silk purse from a sow's ear

You know how it works, remove something, say caffeine or sugar, and the price of the product skyrockets. Mainly because those foods now qualify for the "designer" aisles. In addition, usually the product's weight or volume is decreased.

So, for instance, the 16 oz. pasta for $1.29 becomes the 8 oz. gluten free pasta priced at $4.49 etc. Risking dating myself I can remember the nickel candy bar. It was big and fat. The years rolled by and today that bar is about one-third the size and costs over a dollar.

My frugal nature rebelled immediately. In the name of a test however we sent off for a few of our favorite foods from one internet site and checked out the gluten free sections in each of the two large supermarkets near us. Similar products with different labels for our test. Principally we bought pastas, bread, crackers, chips, pancake mix, baking flour and breakfast cereal. Each of these products on the regular (with gluten) shelves naturally contain wheat and are, item for item less expensive.

The non-packaged foods we buy are fresh produce, lean meat and fish from the ocean (as compared to the fattier farmed-raised fish), eggs, cheese and yogurt.

The gluten free products contained such things as brown rice flour, corn flour, almond flour, flax seed and others but no wheat. No claims to "healthy whole wheat."

Determined not to let this change in diet prove to be boring and out of line with our love of good food, I also began to search out gluten free recipes. I soon realized that damned little would be changed despite the American addiction to wheat and its ubiquitous invasion into nearly everything we have eaten for all of our (unsuspecting) lives.

Yes, I hear the echo of many voices crying for bread. Baguettes, hot dog and hamburger rolls, pumpernickel, crusty French rolls and English muffins. We too love good bread. But what price good health, slim body and organs, a perking brain, and no more cravings or sugar lows?

How many diets have you undertaken that called for compromise? Without giving up something it would not have been a diet. However what I promise you with this diet is an end to the most dangerous enemy to any diet, cravings.

Here is some bad news but far from hopeless. The gluten free bread is not wonderful. Hopefully this will change with demand and an increase in the gluten free population stats. But for French toast, grilled cheese sandwiches, the paninis I make on my waffle iron (why invest in a panini maker if you have a waffle iron? I mean, really) and homemade bread crumbs, it gluten free brown rice bread works just fine. So, sandwiches might be off your menu for now unless you exercise some ingenuity.

I spread mustard and mayonnaise or any spread we are in the mood for onto the bread, shake on maybe some dried basil and lay on some cheddar slices and ham, roast beef, leftover pork, etc. and cook these sandwiches in the large waffle iron. If you already own a panini maker, all the better. The ingredients speak for themselves and the bread shines.

Alternately, we love a large leaf of romaine lettuce wrapped around anything that might go into a sandwich. In fact, in lieu of crackers, rounds of cucumber work fine for dips. What a great way to get more vegetables into your life. There are gluten free wraps however if you really need a sandwich-type meal.

More on food prep just ahead, but first, because it seems always to be on the forefront of my mind, another pep talk.

What has impressed us the most is the change in our attitudes toward food. I was the one who suffered the severe "sugar lows", Ken not so much. I know he is delighted that I no longer suddenly morph into a fire-eating monster when my sugar gets low because I missed a meal or a snack time. But we both realize that meals are now something we eat because we know our bodies need the nourishment. This definitely does not mean that we no longer enjoy our meals but we have completely forgotten to eat lunch on occasion when we are both writing or out and around doing errands. That would never have happened before we went gluten free!

We do look forward to meals because we know that we will enjoy them. I still love cooking and trying new things. In fact, because we both work at home and the hungry lions we used to wake up as have moved we made a morning adjustment. Ken gets up first and makes the coffee. Normally, weekdays he would make three pieces of pumpernickel (one of the highest in gluten breads along with other ryes) for himself and go to his computer. When I got up I made either two medium sized blueberry pancakes or two pieces of toasted seven grain bread for myself. Weekends I cooked eggs, bacon, English muffins and usually garnished the meal with a slice of melon.

Realizing that the hungry lions have departed for good we instituted a weekday morning brunch routine. We work until eleven a.m. at which time we eat either an egg with cheese on top (Ken's favorite) blueberry pancakes, grilled cheese and tomato paninis, or cereal and fruit.

Ken nearly did cartwheels on the deck when he read Dr. Davis's permission to eat eggs and cheese whenever without fear. The opposite of what we had been doing for years.

Nuts are great for us so sometimes I have an almond butter or peanut butter rice cake instead. We enjoy our brunch and return to work until walk time.

Dinner is either pasta with vegetables, olive oil or beef or chicken broth and parmesan cheese. Pasta dishes get more complicated or less depending on what is around. One of my favorite challenges is to dig through what is on hand and make a past meal. Italian red sauce with meatballs topped with grated parmesan always satisfies as does a can of chopped clams added to sautéed mushrooms and chopped red pepper with olive oil and a squirt of lemon juice. The pasta is made with corn or brown rice.

In the past of course there would have been garlic bread. So, add garlic butter and some oregano to the gluten free bread before a quick run under the broiler and thank your lucky stars that it is so darned simple to reclaim your health.

All was going well with our taste and texture tests but meantime, I kept looking for a less expensive way to stick to our new diet. I feel that if a diet is straining your budget then there has to be a better way. That was when I happened upon Vitacost. An on-line shopping experience that is kind to your pocketbook while providing those things you want with something removed, gluten.

There before me were not only all the things we like to eat but at better prices. And believe it or not, the weight and volumes were, in most cases comparable with my former wheat food products. When I tried their all-purpose baking flour I knew the world was back on its proper axis and all would be well.

In addition, if you order a minimum of $49 worth you get free shipping. Stock up and you will be amazed at how much easier it is to create great meals and save money as you glide toward better health.

Going cold turkey (without the bread stuffing)

If you are a busy person, and who isn't these days, save up and invest in a crock-pot (slow cooker) and enjoy home cooked meals ready and waiting for you at the end of your busy day.

It simply does not get any easier than slipping meat, onions, peppers, carrots, cabbage or any combo plus seasonings along with beef or chicken broth, cider or just water into the pot, set it on low, and leave it to do its thing all day. Hold the potatoes to slip in when you get home or they will get too mushy. Pasta or brown rice are also last minute cooking additions to this ready at the end of the day meal. Any hunk of meat, even the lowest price (avoid too much fat) turns delectable in a slow cooker. There is no wheat in this meal like there is in prepared packaged meals aimed at the busy food preparer. Everything about this easy, ready to eat meal it win, win.

If you still need snacks pack cherry tomatoes, cucumber sticks, carrots and to satisfy that old time need, there are great gluten free chips to have with a hunk of cheese. Imagine; once you begin to lose the weight have no guilt about a piece of cheese. As with all good food advice, practice moderation. Satisfy your needs with a small piece of cheese, for instance and eat it very slowly and mindfully.

Now there is a term to add to your daily lexicon. Mindfully. When you begin to really be in the moment as you eat, not reading, watching television or even doing much chatting with a friend and really get into the food, you will move to a higher level of food satisfaction.

Protein is an everyday essential. There is protein in nuts and legumes (beans). We like apple slices spread with peanut butter or a piece of cheese and a small handful of almonds rather than a lunch sandwich. Chickpeas in the chopper with black olives and herb or spice, curry, cumin, basil or oregano, etc. makes a great dip for brown rice chips. We discovered RiceWorks chips and are loving them.

We begin every meal with a salad. We love baby spinach and field greens but they do not keep as well as we'd like. I've decided that they are meant to be eaten immediately and not kept at all. So, I slice cucumbers thin on a mandolin and pile them up under any of combo of tomato slices, avocado chunks, canned beets or corn, zucchini rounds, chopped carrots and apples, purple onions sliced thin on the mandolin, and I make simple vinaigrette dressings. Cole slaw is a favorite. Eat your salad slowly, catch up on the day's news with family, and let those vegetables cheer your body. Speaking of zucchini if you use the insert on the mandolin to make long spaghetti-like strips and quickly cook and cover with Italian red sauce and cheese, you can have dinner on the table in just minutes. Be creative. I know you are busy but meals entered into with little or no mindfulness are no more than shoving in food because you are accustomed to a meal at that time. You eat less when you chew more. You enjoy more when you focus on the food in your mouth rather than the 6 o'clock news.

Stock good extra virgin olive oil, balsamic and other vinegars like red wine vinegar and dried herbs and spices and before you know it, food prep will morph from dumping ingredients out of a cardboard box or popping something frozen into the oven with no mindfulness thus no healthy emotional involvement. If you are going to heal your brain work with it, be mindful and fully there.

Sometimes we would have seconds of a favorite meal. We no longer do because we feel full and satiated with one serving. Do not bring anything into the house that you know you should not eat. Our weakness is ice cream. When it is not there you cannot eat it.

Please do not think that because you go gluten free that all the old rules go out the window with the wheat. They do not. Sensible eating is never out of style.

We love to give small dinner parties for no more than four friends. Our guests are served our diet and so far we have had no complaints albeit we have made some converts. In fact, there is no need to announce that guests are eating gluten free if you are clever about it. The most obvious absence will be the breadbasket however that not need be so if you have time to make a quick bread. Go on-line for gluten free bread recipes and have a ball. Pumpkin and zucchini bread or corn bread with red peppers, onions and cumin are all great. Since anyone can buy bread or dinner rolls you look like the clever hostess by serving up something that is new and exciting.

After you have served that scrumptious no flour chocolate cake with a little whipped cream or strawberries, tell your guests that you just treated them to a body/brain renewal experience. Then you can recommend my book to them.

Staples on hand make cooking easier and more likely to be inventive and interesting. All gluten free, naturally.

Pastas in lots of shapes
Brown Rice
Rice cakes
Burrito shells
Pancake mix and all-purpose baking flour
Chestnut flour makes terrific easy crepes
Canned tomatoes

Canned corn
Canned beets
Tuna
Chopped clams
Red pasta sauce
Kalmata olives
Chickpeas
Black beans
Kidney beans
Bacon (used sparingly chopped in pasta or rice adds a lot of flavor for a small indulgence)
Oils, vinegars, dried herbs and spices.
Lots of fresh produce
Chicken, Pork, Fish, Beef, Lamb
Eggs
Cheeses including a hunk of parmesan or in a jar (real cheese not the phony substitute) for roasted vegetables, pasta etc.

You get the picture. Great meals can come from simple ingredients and although they may not be as quick as processed foods what price health and sanity?

I suggest you read the book that fired me to know more. Cardiologist William Davis M.D.'s Wheat Belly...Lose the Wheat. In addition, you might go to the University of Kansas site on gluten, among other sites. Add up the pros and cons. Go with your gut. Get rid of your gut. Get rid of wheat and gluten and all the problems that come packaged within this grain that constitutes the enemy within.

What have you got to lose but unwanted weight and a really troublesome addiction?

Good luck and happy eating.

Late Breaking News!!!

First, please allow me to apologize for any typos or other goofs as I did not want to take the time to send the manuscript off to my faithful and brilliant proofreader because I simply could not wait to share it with my readers.

Since Ken and I went gluten free three months ago, we have both lost weight, particularly our bellies, lost our cravings, eliminated sugar highs and lows, we eat less and better, and we haven't felt so good in years. Energy, a sharper mind, better sleep, and these are just a few of the changes wrought by our elimination of just one tiny food.

How many times have you investigated a new diet to find that the upheaval to your life, your family's lives, and your bank account would suffer too much if you were to pursue one of those fad diets?

Think about these facts. Wheat is just one type of food that can be ground into flour. Going gluten free does not mean you must give up the enjoyment of eating bread. In fact, by making this change you will discover new ways to add amazingly healthy foods to your diet by adding such things as super-healthy foods like almonds and coconut, avocadoes, antioxidant high berries, cooking oils that actually increase health. Now and then, it is wise to shake up how you have always done some things. When you stress more fresh foods and turn your back forever on processed foods wheat it gone forever. We enjoy a wide variety of home baked breads that are easy on both the baker and the schedule.

Since I wrote this book a great deal of important happenings have taken place regarding GMO's and I cannot, in good conscience, fail to include this current information for my readers.

You will probably read this book too late to take part in the nationwide Occupy Monsanto movement on September 17, however you need to know why they did this if you want to protect your and your loved ones' health and well-being.

Sad to say, while you were still believing that the government food and drug agencies have your best interests at heart, they were instead (as too often is the case in the world and particularly this country) playing footsies with the big mean ogre in the corner of your kitchen waiting to pounce, Monsanto.

Remember how I quoted Monsanto's so honest and straight forward announcements that they gave up their experiments with genetic engineering of such things as wheat and corn in 2004, followed by that heartfelt announcement that there are no genetically modified foods being grown anywhere in the world today? Remember that big fat lie?

Well, the chances are that today you consumed some nice tasty Monsanto-contrived and contaminated food. "Monsanto controls much of the world's food supply at the expense of food democracy worldwide." This from the Occupy Monsanto site. Take a look.

When was the last time you read a label while shopping for groceries only to learn that it was a GMO "food." The quote marks are mine because "Frankenfood" is not real food and people ought only to eat real food. Sure, we as a species are amazingly adaptable. We can and have eaten a wide variety of odd things when really hungry (starving people will try to eat anything that will help them to survive but that does not mean that basic survival and good health are synonymous). Or, maybe when experimenting for whatever reason like when my little sister and I tried eating grass one summer and tossed it up most indelicately on our mother's just washed kitchen floor. Or, when a baby decides to munch on electrical wires, or the silly puppy takes an interest in eating stones. But when it comes right down to it, the best way to stay healthy is to eat real, healthy food.

Okay, back to the original inquiry. When was the last time you read a label clearly posted on a food saying that it is made from GMO's or, genetically modified organisms? The answer is NEVER because Monsanto (and others, you insert here who you think might have no conscience about what the American public ingests) have made sure you do not know that well-protected secret.

Congress gave Monsanto and other unethical agribusiness scientists a nice slippery loophole to slide through on that score. "Hey, it's still wheat (corn, etc.) so no need to label it." In addition, because it is "still" whatever the food might be, what it always has been, no need to do studies on humans just to make sure that it is "still" what it purports to be. How do you feel about being a guinea pig for your government food advisors and so-called experts on nutrition? I, for one, am damned furious about the matter.

Monsanto shells out $4.2 million to stop GMO labeling law

This from examiner.com. Check it out. The gist of it is that the fight is on over genetically modified food. In California, Monsanto is out to squash like a bug under it's unethical boot, Proposition 37, a GMO labeling law set to hit the ballots on Election Day November 2012. The agribusiness firm Monsanto just put up $4.2 million to ensure that the measure is defeated and GMO labels stay off our food. Who are the bad guys here? They do not need to wear special hats to be quickly identified.

But Monsanto is not alone. Other biotech giants like Dupont Pioneer and Cargill have amassed $25 million to run negative ads in advance of November's GMO vote. Naturally, the good guys do not have the financial clout to fight the battle on an even playing ground: Pro-labeling advocates, in contrast, have raised only $2.4 million. David has a big stick, and Goliath has a stealth bomber. Oh, goodie.

Don't you just get sick of being lied to from the top down? I do.

Then there are the big bad wolf scare tactics like this, also from examiner.com.

Opponents of the bill, however, are quick to tell consumers (that) labeling food will mean higher prices at the grocery store. "Everyone is impacted because everyone buys groceries, and one of the impacts is going to be higher grocery bills," Kathy Fairbanks said, speaking for the No on 37, a campaign funded largely by agribusiness dollars.

Walmart To Sell Unlabeled GMO Corn From Monsanto

"At prices this low, how could you expect the food not to be laced with insecticide?" Russia Today reports.

"The retail giant says they won't advertise which of their products are made with genetically modified organisms, or GMOs." This from a site called disinformation.com.

Want more?

"We've gone on at great lengths discussing the dangers of genetic modification. Monsanto's GMO corn has been linked to weight gain and organ function disruption, while GMO crops and pesticides destroy our farmland and environment." From EDUCATION NEWS.

There's a story doing the rounds again about how Monsanto, one of the world's largest profiteers of genetically engineered (GE) food, banned GE food from its own corporate canteens!

"Monsanto had its pants pulled down by Friends of the Earth in 1999, who revealed that the company was refusing to serve to its own staff the very same GE food that it incessantly foists upon impoverished nations on the premise that it will save populations from starvation. Although it has never been proved, Monsanto constantly claims that GE food is harmless – so why wasn't it serving it in its own office?

"In one canteen, run by external provider, Sutcliffe Catering, a notice read that a decision has been taken to remove, as far as practicable, GE soya and maize from all food products served in the canteen. "We have taken the above steps to ensure that you, the customer, can feel confident in the food we serve, the provider said." Greenpeace

Are you as upset as I am about the terrible news over the collapse in bee colonies world-wide from insecticides?

Here is a nugget from EUCATION NEWS.

"Amid all the controversy over genetically-modified (GM) crops and their pesticides and herbicides decimating bee populations all around the world, biotechnology behemoth Monsanto has decided to buy out one of the major international firms devoted to studying and protecting bees. According to a company announcement, Beeologics handed over the reins to Monsanto back on September 28, 2011, which means the gene-manipulating giant will now be able to control the flow of information and products coming from Beeologics for colony collapse disorder (CCD)."

The Huffington Post Green site reporter Michelle Simon posted the top ten lies from Monsanto coming up to Proposition 37 in

California. For instance: "The safety and benefits of these ingredients are well established."

Michelle goes on to explain why this is an outright lie. Unfortunately, no long-term studies exist on either the safety or benefits of GMO ingredients, so Monsanto has no basis for making such a claim. Indeed, the U.S. Food and Drug Administration does not even require safety studies of genetically engineered foods. Meanwhile, some independent studies raise questions about links to allergies and other potential health risks.

In the final analysis, only you can be the judge of whom to trust and who is lying to the American public about the dangers present in what we all eat. All the information is out there if you have the time to seek it out.

One way to avoid eating genetically modified organisms is to avoid eating wheat to begin with. Unfortunately, until the government stops allowing GMOs on the market with no testing for reactions to these foods by the human body, this is a tricky road to travel. However, the jury is in about the effect genetic engineering has had on the gluten content of wheat and it is not good. So, you can take a giant step right now and make your own bread from the large variety of other flours that are not wheat. I make my own bread both by hand and bread machine using the "other" great flours like coconut, almond, corn, chickpea, rice, etc. Just because you cannot eat wheat flour does not mean you must give up bread, pancakes, French toast, croutons, cookies, cake, pies, biscotti, etc. Yes, the joys of eating flour-based foods continues on even after you give up wheat flour.

Stick to fresh produce, brown rice, rice or corn pastas, organic chicken and pork, beef in moderation, fish that wild and not farmed, and check all products for the addition of wheat that is amazingly insidious in so many foods. Treat packaged, quickie foods like they are contaminated with plague germs. Think fresh, and when you can, buy organic. It is not a perfect scheme, but it is better than what has been making us all unhealthy since science was allowed, and supported in its efforts, to do us all dirt by changing Mother Nature's perfect balance of chromosomes and genes in wheat, etc. into a dangerous "Frankenfood."

Next time you and your loved ones break bread together make it a nice hearty loaf of, say, cheddar herb almond flour bread or coconut cinnamon rice bread.

Bon appetit!

2013 Up-date

When I wrote this book, initially, Monsanto had yet to be given carte blanche, a green light, the go-ahead of all go-aheads to poison our food with impunity.

In early 2013, a legislative rider was inserted into the Senate Continuing Resolution spending bill that was deceptively disguised under the title Farmer Assurance Provision. Sec.

735 of this bill "grants Monsanto the immunity from federal courts pending the review of any GM crop that is thought to be dangerous.

This means that the federal courts have been rendered impotent with regard to stopping Monsanto from continuing to plant GM crops, even should the U.S. government itself determine them to be a danger to either the environment or human health.

It was the machinations of Roy Blunt Republican Senator from Missouri who colluded with Monsanto to write the Monsanto Protection Act. As it were, Monsanto wrote its own protection act that is tight as a drum and gives them full license to endanger the environment and human lives with Genetically Engineered foods. In addition, to put a stinking frosting on their cake, they are now also free to kill us through other insidious means.

The people who brought us Agent Orange, and more recently, Roundup pesticide, and who now call themselves a GREEN COMPANY are fully enabled, in perpetuity, to continue their farmer-indentured-servant plan of God-like control over the seeds, fertilizer, and pesticides used by farmers in their agribusiness block.

Some countries have wised up. Poland, for one, has made unlawful the planting of any GMO seeds until, or if, the time ever comes when they GMO crops are proved safe for human consumption.

When a government chooses to serve (and be controlled by) corporations over people, that Rome has definitely begun its descent into complete collapse. Corporations do not eat these dangerous crops...people do, however.

Acknowledgments and Credits

William Davis M.D.
Oxford American Dictionary
Wikipedia
University of Kansas
Dr. Tom Hyman
U.S. Dept. of Agriculture
ChooseMyPlate.gov
Dorothy Parker
benatlas.com
David Kirkpatrick's blog on technology
PubMed Health
Dr. Jay Adlersburg
Natural Health School
Fat Head Blog Tom Naughton
Easy Health Options
Insulite Lab
Huffington Post
EDUCATION NEWS
Occupy Monsanto
Greenpeace

Cynthia Gallant-Simpson earned degrees in Psychology and Holistic health from Lesley College, Cambridge, MA. As an exchange student in England at Ealing College, near London, she studied Abnormal Psychology and enjoyed a lecture course called Anatomy of the British Mystery Genre.

She began her writing career as a journalist for a small, south of Boston, daily newspaper. From there, because she and her husband are dedicated sailors, she moved on to writing sailing, cruising and galley provisioning and recipe articles for U.S. and Canada cruising and live aboard magazines.

She is the author of numerous adult mysteries, illustrated children's books, two chapter books for middle readers and her beloved (British-style) cozy mysteries. Her books are available on Amazon and Kindle.

In 2005, she and her husband sold their antique sea captain's house on Cape Cod, sold or gave away to family everything not required for living on a forty-four foot boat and moved aboard.

With friends and family still on Cape Cod, their summer "home" is their boat moored in Pleasant Bay. Winters are spent in warmer climes.

She is gluten free, has lost her post-menopausal belly everyone told her was just part of ageing, no longer has sugar lows or cravings, eats less and enjoys it more and has more energy and a clearer mind than when wheat was her enemy within.